Outpatient Psychiatry

Psychiatric Outpatient Centers of America (POCA) is an organization of Psychiatric Clinics and Community Mental Health Centers in the United States, Canada, and Mexico. It was founded in 1963. Some of its many purposes have been to: disseminate information of importance to its clinic membership, offer consultative services to new and established agencies, organize forums for discussing mutual professional and administrative problems, make available group insurance plans for member clinics as well as other group benefits, publish lasting literature in the field and a newsletter covering current information relative to legislation, etc. POCA holds an annual spring meeting that provides much of the material presented in these volumes. Though special services of POCA are available only to member clinics, the annual meeting is open to all interested professionals and nonprofessionals.

For further information contact:

HAROLD WERNER, ACSW
101 Harter Road
Morristown, NJ 07969

Outpatient Psychiatry:

Progress, Treatment, Prevention

Edited by
ROBERT E. KOGAN
JOHN T. SALVENDY

POCA Perspectives No. 9

The University of Alabama Press

Library of Congress Cataloging in Publication Data

Main entry under title:

Outpatient psychiatry.

(POCA perspectives; no. 9)
Modified versions of papers presented at 2 annual
meetings of POCA, held in 1979 and 1980.
Includes bibliographical references.
1. Psychiatric hospitals—Outpatient services—
Congresses. 2. Psychiatric clinics—Congresses.
3. Community mental health services—Congresses.
I. Kogan, Robert E., 1937–   . II. Salvendy, John T.,
1937–   . III. Psychiatric Outpatient Centers of
America. IV. Series. [DNLM: 1. Mental disorders—
Therapy—Congresses. 2. Community mental health
services—Congresses. W1 P658 no. 9 / WM30 094]
RC439.2.097   1985   616.89   83-6911
ISBN 0-8173-0171-2

To
MICHAEL DINOFF

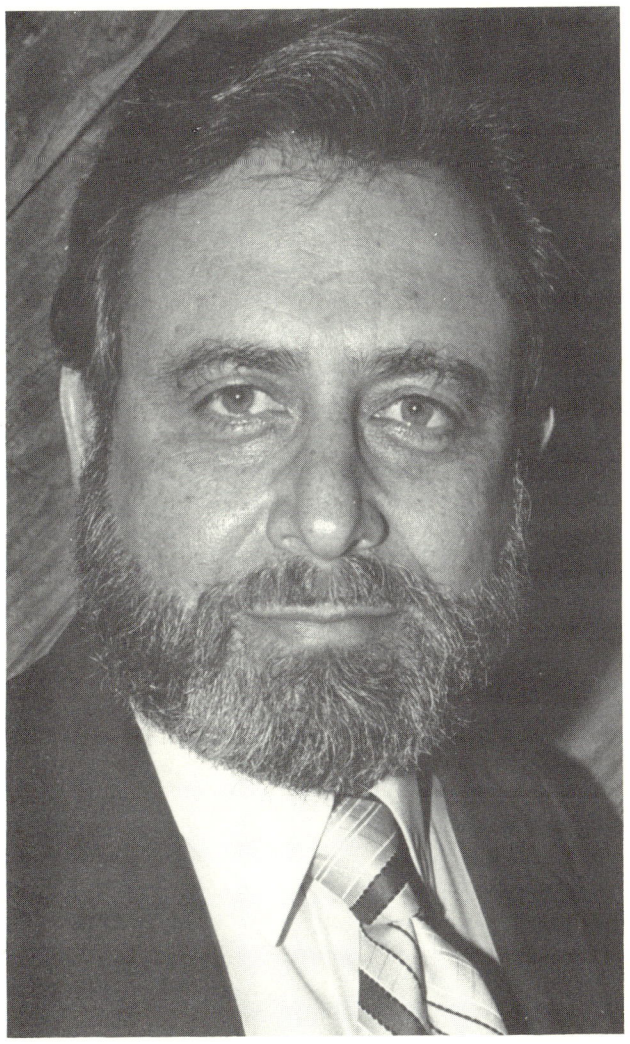

PHOTO BY BETH DINOFF

Contents

Dedication

To dedicate a volume to a close friend is not an easy task. Subjective feelings tend to mingle with objective fact. And yet, when speaking of Michael Dinoff, everyone who knew him understood how much his person was bound up in everything he did. His sudden death has deprived the psychological and academic community, as well as POCA and his friends, of a person whose warmth and dedication filled every task he undertook and every relationship he had.

A product of New York City where he was born in 1933, Mike completed his undergraduate studies at Indiana University. His interest was always in the area of psychology, and, after completing work on a master's degree at The University of Alabama, he earned a doctorate at the University of Tennessee in 1960. In 1953 he married, and he is survived by his wife, Sandy, and his three children.

Mike's involvement in the professional community was always multi-faceted. At the time of his death he served as Professor and Director of the Psychological Clinic at The University of Alabama. At the same time he served as Administrative Director of the B'nai Brith Hillel Foundation of Tuscaloosa, acted as consultant to Birmingham-Southern College and Medfit, and was a senior Professional Consultant with our firm, Reed and Di Salvo Associates of New York City. He had a variety of experience with the Veterans Administration, in research, in consultation with business, and in clinical practice.

As part of his professional commitment to the community at large Mike, at one time or another, served as consultant to more than twenty groups and organizations. These included the American School in Madrid, the National Council on the Elderly and the Department of Defense. He served on several academic and legislative committees and edited a variety of journals. He was very much involved in some of the landmark mental health legislation in Alabama during the past decade.

Throughout his career Mike remained active in professional organizations. He was a fellow of the American Psychological Association and a Diplomate of the ABPP. He served as President of the Alabama Psychological Association and of POCA. In 1982 he was the recipient of The University of Alabama Alumni Association's "Outstanding Commitment to Teaching Award."

In his busy schedule Mike also found time to write. Either alone or in conjunction with colleagues he wrote over forty articles and research papers. These addressed issues in psychotherapy, interviewing, varieties of behavior, and behavior modification. For the past several years he served as permanent editor for the POCA Proceedings. The editorship was time consuming and detailed in its demands; Mike's ability to synthesize material and the varied styles of different authors was a key factor in providing continuity and consistent quality for the series of volumes published.

His relationship to POCA covered more than a decade. My first contact with Mike was when I invited him to present a paper at the annual meeting held in San Francisco. He was asked to serve on the board of directors and in the years following served POCA as Treasurer, Vice-President, and President. In 1977 he planned and directed the annual meeting held in New Orleans, the theme focusing on "Neglected Services—Children and the Elderly."

No simple recitation of his contributions and accomplishments can in any way provide a full profile of Michael Dinoff. To those of us who knew him well and worked with him his energy, compassion, and willingness to engage both task and person were attributes that made him special.

We had the opportunity of working together on a variety of consulting assignments over the years. Frequently we would take long walks together—often early in the morning. We shared our personal and professional concerns, our humor, our sadness, our joys and disappointments. Mike's understanding and support was always warm and genuine. His questions and interpretations were accomplished with sensitivity and respect, and any suggestions he had to make were made with compassion. He was present with his whole being—a sign of love and concern that one does not often see. And this is how Michael Dinoff approached everyone he met, everyone he knew, and everyone he worked with.

Reading back over what I have written I cannot help but feel that there are many facts that have not been included and many feelings that have not been expressed. But in trying to draw a profile of this particular man that would always be the feeling, no matter how many words were written.

It is, I suppose, sufficient and appropriate, simply to dedicate this volume to the memory of Michael Dinoff, a deeply involved and respected professional, a sincere and concerned human being, and a beloved friend.

CHARLES DI SALVO, Ph.D.
New York City

In Memoriam

Michael Dinoff, an exceptional clinical psychologist, was born in and grew up in New York City. In 1953 he married the former Sondra Miselson, whom he had known most of his life. Together with their two daughters and one son, the Dinoffs created a welcome home atmosphere which, over the years, they shared fully with friends, students, and others in need of caring and personal support. He received a B.A. degree from Indiana University in 1955 and, continuing to pursue his interest in psychology, an M.A. degree from The University of Alabama in 1957. Three years later he earned his Ph.D. degree from the University of Tennessee and began his distinguished career as a clinical psychologist. His views of psychology were particularly influenced by Paul S. Siegel at Alabama and by Gerald R. Pascal and W. O. Jenkins at Tennessee.

He was appointed an Assistant Professor in the Psychology Department of The University of Alabama in 1963 where he remained throughout his career, achieving rapid promotions through the professorial ranks based upon his high level of research productivity, outstanding teaching, administrative skills, and contributions to the University and profession. Throughout most of that period he directed the department's Psychological Clinic, demanding of that facility an excellence that was consonant with his own personal standards as a clinical psychologist. He believed that a clinical professor should model for students the highest level of professional attainment and to that end obtained licensure, diplomate standing, and fellowships in relevant divisions of the American Psychological Association. He consulted numerous groups and professional organizations and served as an officer for a variety of associations and boards. He was particularly proud of his association with and services to the Organization of Psychiatric Outpatient Centers of America. Of his extensive list of research publications, none were more important to him than the edited series reporting their proceedings.

Michael Dinoff will be remembered as a warm, outgoing person who could be described as charismatic in the best sense of the word. His humor was sharp but never sarcastic or mean. If he had something to say, he said it straight out. Clearing the air was important to Mike, and he did a lot of it. He loved people—family, colleagues, clients, students, and community. He was a friend with great clinical empathy and a therapist who knew how to be a friend. He felt personal responsibility for others and gave freely of his energy and large store of knowledge. His death from an apparent heart attack occurred May 17, 1982, following a characteristically unselfish act— an afternoon community solicitation for a fund drive. We shall miss him.

CHARLES L. RICKARD

Preface

The themes in this volume are modified versions of papers presented at the Seventeenth and Eighteenth Annual International Meetings of the Association of Psychiatric Outpatient Centers of America (POCA). The aim of the editors has been to present to students, practitioners, and researchers in the field of mental health a selection of writings reflecting the state of the art on the verge of the 1980s. In the tradition of previous POCA Proceedings, the emphasis has been on presenting either innovative approaches to mental health care delivery or authoritative reviews of specific treatment modalities and techniques. While no single book can claim today to describe comprehensively the developments in outpatient psychiatry, we think that POCA Perspectives Number Nine complements well the gaps left by contemporary textbooks and handbooks.

In editing this book we have tried to do justice to the memory of our friend, colleague, and longtime coeditor of the POCA Perspectives, Mike Dinoff, Ph.D., who passed away unexpectedly while working on this volume.

R.K.
J.T.S.

POCA awards to:

WAYNE D. HOLTZMAN, Ph.D.
Recipient, Tenth Annual Award

HEINZ LEHMANN, M.D.,
Recipient, Eleventh Annual Award

Previous Recipients:

Gisela Konopka, D.S.W.
Fritz Redl, Ph.D.
Gerald Kaplan, M.D.
Rollo May, Ph.D.
Hon. William O. Douglas
Erich Lindemann, Ph.D., M.D.
Leo Kanner, M.D.
Theodore Lidz, M.D.
Leopold Bellak, M.D.

Part I:
Community Mental Health:
Change, Transition, or Crisis?

Foreword to Part I

Robert E. Kogan, M.A.

The theme of the Seventeenth Annual International Meeting of the Association of Psychiatric Outpatient Centers of America was "Community Mental Health: Change, Transition, or Crisis?" Long before such terms as "Block Grant Funding," "New Federalism," and "Reaganomics" became part of our everyday vocabulary, mental health professionals were acutely aware of pending changes on the horizons. While the nation was preparing for massive political and economic changes, mental health centers were failing to meet the challenge of the 1960s to establish a "bold new approach" to mental health. Centers throughout the United States were closing due to bankruptcy, poor administration, poor or no accountability, and inability to provide appropriate services to the highest community priority—its chronically mentally ill. While most mental health centers emulated the private practice model, the leadership within the field demanded change. Advocates of both the Mental Health Systems Act and the Balanced Service System were attempting to create a more responsive system of mental health care, based on providing services to the chronically mentally ill in the least restrictive environment, which would be built on the assets and strengths of the consumers and their support system. The Seventeenth Annual International Meeting of POCA attempted to address these issues. Change was imminent. No one knew what direction it would take, but its results would soon be measured in terms of quality care or chaos.

Some of the more important workshops during this annual meeting were: (1) Prevention and Rehabilitation: Our Neglected Priorities; (2) Federal Funding for Mental Health—New Directions and Legislation; (3) Deinstitutionalization: Community Programs for the Chronic; (4) Intake Assessment: Levels of Functioning and Role Performance; (5) Accreditation of Mental Health Centers by the Joint Commission on Accreditation of Hospitals; (6) Clinical Role of Religion; (7) Peer

3

Review: A Constructive Process or a Kangaroo Court? (8) Optimum Clinical Environment: Hospital? University? Private Practice? Natural Environment? (9) Concerns and Issues Involving a Board of Directors and Their Relationship to Staff; and (10) The Role of a Mental Health Center in the Aftermath of Natural Disasters.

Many of the papers contained in this book are a result of this annual meeting. These topics are as relevant now as they were then.

Acknowledgments

The author would like to express his love and appreciation to Dr. Michael Dinoff for his help and assistance in the organization of the Seventeenth Annual International Meeting of POCA, and for his friendship and encouragement throughout the years. The author would also like to thank Jane Davenport Starrett, President of the Board of Directors of the New Horizons Mental Health Center for her continued encouragement and support in having this book published.

De-institutionalization of the Mentally Ill: Expectations, Reality, and Future Outlook

John T. Salvendy, M.D.

De-institutionalization is a process involving the shunning or avoidance of traditional institutional settings, primarily mental hospitals, *and* a concurrent expansion of community-based services for the treatment of the mentally ill (10). Where, how, and at what cost will a community accommodate its emotionally handicapped members has been repeatedly in the center of heated discussion for the past two centuries. However, the problems involved are not yet historical. Again, our society is at crossroads on this issue.

Two decades ago, well-meaning and enthusiastic professionals and ambitious politicians joined hands to give birth to a Utopian mental health system, which was to humanize (again) the treatment of chronic psychiatric patients. The expectations raised were high, yet the preceeding research to substantiate cause and effect links was woefully inadequate. Patients' views and attitudes of the public were not explored and the expected benefits for both groups were only hypothesized and often were in the form of wishful thinking.

After having the process of de-institutionalization tested over the past decade and a half, a definite sobering has occurred in mental health circles. Some of the positive effects of de-institutionalization have been demonstrated early in the process. Recently critical reviews and evaluations have prevailed. After having scanned the balance sheet, both the governmental agencies and the mental health professionals seem to agree (though not always publicly, for face-saving reasons) that significant changes will have to occur in the field of comprehensive aftercare for psychiatric patients if the original

5

intentions are to materialize. These changes will be necessary, not only in order to avoid a further demoralization of both patients and staff, but also in order to help the governments at all levels to plan and evolve realistic and viable treatment modifications and alternatives. The fate of the de-institutionalized patient has been closely linked with the availability of a community-based network of support systems. In most instances the "king-pin" in that system has been the local mental health center. Owing to its historical role in the development of extramural services and to the volume of rhetoric, hope, and finances committed to this institution, the community mental health center concept will receive a thorough analysis here.

The other emphasis will be on understanding the historical background leading to the concept of de-institutionalization of the mentally ill. At this stage of our sociopolitical development, we cannot afford to reinvent the wheel every couple of generations! The issues at stake are too crucial—the psychological and fiscal investment are of such magnitude that we must not allow for more blunders. We should try to learn from past experiences and anticipate new ones, so that we will not be forced to throw out the baby with the bath water!

The purpose of this paper is to analyze the psychosocial, pharmacological, ethical, and political developments leading up to the present state of de-institutionalization. Further, a critical appraisal of past and present influential philosophies will be carried out, along with an assessment of the impact of the programs already available. An attempt will be made to recommend certain measures to ameliorate the situation.

The observations and comments in this paper were derived from the following sources: a review of the international literature, with a particular emphasis on sociohistorical developments, pharmacotherapy, psychosocial treatment, existing programs, evaluation research, political-fiscal issues, and staff problems; my experience as Director of the Psychiatric Out-patient Services at St. Michael's Hospital, University of Toronto (since 1975) and as the coordinator for Community Psychiatric Services (since 1971) at the same facility (which is a teaching general hospital in a downtown metropolitan area, with a large chronic mentally ill population); my participation as a founding Vice-President of Community Resources Consultants (1973–1976), an Ontario government-financed "super agency"

("Service-for-Services") designed for planning, integration, coordination, stimulation, and evaluation of aftercare facilities for psychiatric patients in Metropolitan Toronto; visiting, teaching, and working in a large number of mental health facilities in North America, Western and Eastern Europe, and Israel.

Background

In Antiquity and the Middle Ages, the mentally ill were perceived as afflicted by bad spirits. At times they were ascribed prophetic qualities or were seen as possessed by the devil (144). Their communities either tolerated them, tried to exorcise them, or hunted them as witches. With the advent of secularism and the waning of the church's power in the eighteenth century, these individuals were perceived as social deviants who showed "moral turpitude." At this time institutionalization started to replace witch hunting (11), but it was devised more to protect society than to look after the patient's well-being. Incarceration in these early asylums was a most degrading, inhumane experience. Descriptions from reformers such as Pinel, Pritchard, Rush, Connolly, Griesinger, and others (26, 38, 45, 53, 67, 91, 95, 103, 105, 107, 113, 144) sound appalling. Many patients were chained for years. Food and lighting were inadequate and practically no treatment was provided.

It was not until the ascendency of "moral treatment" as advocated by the previously mentioned innovators and Dorothea Dix in the first third of the nineteenth century that a more humane approach to the treatment of the mentally ill was developed. An increasing medical understanding of the nature and causes of bizarre behavior led to its acceptance as an illness rather than a sinister social deviance.

After a few small mental hospitals were built in a number of countries, the efforts of dedicated lay people and professionals (such as Dorothea Dix, Pinel, Connolly, and others) in the second half of the nineteenth century led to the building of numerous asylums in the true sense, both by their respective governments and by private enterprise (2, 38, 45, 53, 67, 79, 91, 95, 103, 119, 122, 136, 144). These institutions were frequently erected away from population centers. More often than not they had a wall around their compounds, and the patients were usually segregated from other people, including their relatives. However, even this modest achievement in a more humane tradition did not last long. In North America primarily through mass immigration and in Europe through decreasing mortality rates, the asylums became overcrowded. Patient care deteriorated and both the psychiatrists and the public lost faith in the possibility for cure and reintegration in the community (11). With a few exceptions (79, 144) by the early twentieth century, the large state mental hospitals were bogged down in bureaucratic morass and financial difficulties. Patients were incarcerated, were given little care, and were frequently abused.

With few exceptions this situation lasted well into the period of the Second World War. The overwhelming majority of the mentally ill were treated intramurally for months, years, and often decades. The effects of this long-term hospitalization in huge, isolated, impersonal settings, both on patients and staff, were colorfully depicted from the late forties on in a number of now classic studies. Bettelheim and Sylvester talked of a rigid, noncaring regime that allowed no room for individual decisions and demanded only compliance from patients. It led to emotional apathy, lack of spontaneity and motivation, and an incapacity for active adjustment (14). Wing has described the end result in terms of an absence of interest, resignation, dependence, depersonalization, and reliance on fantasy. These are the hallmarks of *institutionalism*, a pattern of behavior that is evoked in an individual by the social pressures of an institution (140).

Goffman labeled such segregated communities (which also include prisons, tuberculosis sanitaria, orphanages, prisoner-of-war camps, refugee camps, etc.) as "total institutions" and listed a number of features which they have in common: the staff and inmates have fundamentally different points of view and often perceive each other in narrow, hostile stereotypical roles. There is great social distance between the two sides (i.e., staff and inmates) and little intermixing. Decisions about admission and discharge are made by authority, and the individual has little say in them. The amount of extramural contact is strictly rationed and is perceived as a privilege. All social, therapeutic, and vocational activity is rigidly regimented, and the patient's ability to perform everyday roles atrophies through the lack of use, as his contact with the outside world is reduced to a minimum (12, 21, 48, 49, 54, 116, 117, 140). Moreover, the understanding of the effects of "total institutions" has helped us separate symptoms that were primarily attributed to the illness per se from those caused by the long incarceration.

In addition, Ellenberger and Wing have described a group, primarily composed of chronic schizophrenics, who seem to have a particular susceptibility to rapid institutionalism, and thus the problem is aggravated even more (41, 140). Because of their preponderance among the chronic patient population of mental hospitals, the problem of institutionalism has been to a large measure tantamount to the problem of the long-term management of schizophrenia.

In response to this criticism, public opinion and governmental sources realized that regardless of the original humane intentions, these institutions were not fulfilling their tasks adequately anymore, i.e., certainly not in a way commensurate with present social climate and the potential implied in numerous studies. The impression was that these settings became not only inhumane and ineffective, but also through the long detention policies too inefficient. In the late fifties the need arose to develop alternatives to incarceration and institutionalism (78). Corresponding to this social-political development and equally important in its impact upon the de-institutionalization of the emotionally ill has been the introduction of the first major tranquilizers and anti-depressants in the mid-fifties. As these two evolutions occurred almost concommitantly and influenced each other's effect reciprocally on the mentally ill, attempts for a separate and independent evaluation of their respective roles in diminishing inpatient populations have been difficult to design and implement.

The Effects of Pharmacotherapy

The need to use mood-altering drugs has been recognized in the civilizations of the ancient Middle East and Greece. In the Middle Ages their formal use decreased (aside from that of alcohol) in Europe owing to the dangerous misconception that people who saw things differently were possessed by demons and thus were best eliminated.

Opiates and their derivatives have thrived, though, for centuries longer in the Middle East, the Orient, and South America. In Western Europe the scientific study of psychoactive drugs had not started until the mid nineteenth century. Bromides were used for decades with the notion that they had a beneficial effect on the supposedly excited central nervous system of the mental patient. The first drugs that achieved a lasting popularity almost to our day were the barbiturates, developed in Germany at the turn of the century. At first the rationale for their use was similar to the one attributed to the bromides (2). Later they were abused further as hypnotica. Prior to and during World War II, amphetamines were used in the treatment of depression and in order to cope with overtiredness (for the crews of German warplanes and tanks). They were later abandoned because of troublesome side effects and aftereffects.

Chlorpromazine, the first major tranquilizer was introduced by Delay and Deniker in France in the early 1950s. At the same time reserpine was introduced into the treatment of depression (34). On the North American continent, Heinz Lehmann pioneered the introduction of psychotropic drugs into the treatment of the mentally ill. The fast-spreading use of phenothiazines and other drugs that came later has revolutionized the treatment of psychotic patients, schizophrenics in particular. The ubiquitous use of these relatively safe drugs has greatly contributed to the reduction in the number of patients in mental hospitals and drastically shortened the duration of their stay. This development has allowed the focus to shift from institutional therapy to community-based follow-up programs (85). A number of studies in the United States and Europe have since documented this dramatic transformation of treatment results and its impact on the mental hospital populations (1, 85, 94, 100, 128, 131).

Furthermore, Mosher pointed out that the success of psychopharmacological treatment had a significant indirect effect on the socialtherapeutic scene as well (96). The stigma of untreatability having been removed, professionals and politicians alike felt more comfortable to experiment with more humane, democratic, and communityoriented programs for chronic schizophrenics. The beneficiaries were not just the individual patients and their families. The "total institutions" could now opt for a more participatory, active treatment-oriented approach, without having to stress too much their custodian roles.

This discussion is not to say that the psychotropic revolution has not had its share of problems and criticism. The use of psychoactive drugs generates controversy in some circles, as no consensus has been reached on how and who should control what kind of socially deviant behavior. However, this task seems to be beyond the scope of the mental health field. The solutions required are as much social, political, and ethical as they are professional. This controversy does not mean that we should withdraw, but we should not pretend that we can and want to make decisions that are outside our jurisdiction!

The Psychosocial Changes

Chronologically, the psychosocial revolution in the field of psychiatric treatment has preceded the advent of psychopharmacology. However, its expansion has been parallel to the latter for the past two and a half decades. This development had a long history. As early as the beginning of this century Adolf Meyer called for services of a collaborative nature in the community (90). Kraepelin recommended more than sixty years ago that in order to educate the public, it was important to establish "patient-advocate" style groups and to promote communication and contacts between the staffs of asylums and the community. He vocally supported the notion of sheltered work situations, along with the boarding of the chronic patients with their families or in foster homes under medical supervision (79). A community-based management of mental patients has been practiced for a thousand years in the village of Gheel in Belgium (144).

After the Second World War the impact of the sociological studies such as Goffman's (49) and Stanton and Schwarz's (130) describing the deleterious effects of long-term hospitalization started to affect both the set-up of the mental hospitals themselves and a shift to extramural facilities. At the same time, the British experimented with the "open hospital" system. Concomitantly Bierer established the first therapeutic social clubs for former psychiatric patients (15). Moreover Maxwell Jones's development of the concept of therapeutic community (71) has injected further optimism into this field. Yet it was not until the introduction of psychoactive drugs in the mid 1950s that both professionals and the public at large were willing to experiment on a larger scale. At that stage the functioning of mental hospitals started to evolve along more therapeutic lines. A decrease in social distance between patients and staff was fostered along with better communication among the different professional groups to improve staff morale. From the late 1950s forward, the psychiatric establishment and the public were ready to consider specific alternatives to inhospital treatment.

These trends have prompted the British government to promulgate the Mental Health Act, 1959 (115) and the American Congress to establish in 1955 a Joint Commission on Mental Illness and Health. This Commission evaluated the state of mental health care delivery and delineated by 1960 recommendations for a national mental health program (70). This groundwork formed the core of the now historical legislation brought in by President John F. Kennedy as the "Mental Retardation Facilities and Community Mental Health Centers Construction Act of 1963" (73). The intent of both of these enactments and later amendments was to shift the focus in the treatment of the mentally ill from the large, frequently remote and isolated institutions to the local community. It was expected to prevent admissions to a hospital of any sort by offering comprehensive outpatient services.

The idea of community mental health suggested a twofold promise: management of the emotionally ill within the community and the promotion of mental health in general. The community in this context should not be too narrowly defined, because it means different things according to the setting. It can be seen geographically, jurisdictionally (as a neighborhood in the city, county, state, region, etc.) or as a population of a limited size in relationship to location (i.e., "catchment area"). It can also be a community of interest for the common cause. Hume offers a functional definition of the community as a system of systems where the intergovernmental, interagency, interprofessional, interpersonal, and administrator-consumer relationships are viewed as essential to the initiation, development, and effective utilization of all available resources for remedial and rehabilitative measures in the field of mental health (68).

In order to fulfil the requirements of a community-oriented approach, a proper infrastructure of extensive support systems had to be created. These systems were to offer comprehensive and coordinated treatment and rehabilitative services. Inherent in this conceptualization was the hope that mental illness could be prevented and that even chronic patients could be reintegrated into society at large. The mass media played an equivocal role in an attempt to change age-old fears and prejudices. As an indicator of increasing acceptance and hopefulness, the number of psychiatric inpatient and outpatient departments mushroomed in the general hospitals.

The psychiatric profession itself was among the initiators of change. Although some, such as T. Szasz and R. D. Laing, tended to make the point through the approach of "overkill," the movement toward a liberalization of custody and treatment philosophies accelerated markedly from the mid-fifties on. This trend toward a more community-based treatment and comprehensive aftercare brought with it a rapid expansion and involvement of other mental health professionals, such as social workers, psychologists, occupational therapists, public health nurses, administrators, and lay volunteer community workers.

This evolution had a number of political and fiscal aspects as well. A variety of civil rights' groups became very active in representing patients' interests, both in and outside the hospitals. Their vocal lobbying frequently affected the direction and purpose of a number of legislative acts although not always in the best interest of the patient's treatment. Such was the case with the United States Congress Community Mental Health Centers Act of 1963 (137) and its several amendments along with the Canadian Hastings Report (59) and the last amendment to the Ontario Mental Health Act of 1978 (133).

The introduction of universal and comprehensive health care insurance, including all forms of psychiatric treatment, in Canada over a decade ago and its anticipated implementation in the near future in the United States are further indicators of the growing understanding (however tenuous at times) that the mentally ill should have equal rights in regard to treatment (32). This notion found its crystalization in the willingness of all three levels of government, i.e., federal, state, and municipal, to contribute financially to the planning, development, maintenance, and evaluation of community mental health programs.

The Theory and Practice of Extramural Care

The basis for a conceptualization of out-of-institution care was provided by the federal Mental Health Centers Program requirements. The minimal essential services to be provided had to include inpatient care, outpatient care, emergency services on a twenty-four hour basis, partial hospitalization, and community consultation and education. Furthermore it was recommended that an additional five services be provided by such community based centers: precare and aftercare for patients hospitalized in long-term care settings, diagnostic facilities, rehabilitative services, research and evaluation programs, and arrangements for training and education (137). The community to be served has been defined usually in terms of a geographic catchment area. Its size has optimally varied between 75,000 and 200,000 with allowances for reasonable exceptions. It has been felt that a program serving a population of less than 75,000 would not be economically viable, while a community over 200,000 would be too large for effective and coordinated interagency cooperation. Levenson noted that the emphasis in these programs has been on secondary prevention (that is, the reduction of prevalence by early and active treatment of the illness) along with tertiary prevention (the reduction of residual disabilities through rehabilitation and aftercare). He pointed out that primary prevention, or consultative and educational services to the community, has been neglected. It happened because of the unfamiliarity of many professionals with this concept and because of fiscal restraints (86). This limited emphasis on prevention is furthermore directly related to the difficulty of marshaling replicable evidence as to the efficacy and cost effectiveness of this approach.

The first practical step in the organization of community programs is that of fact-finding (25, 68). The basic guidelines for the establishment and maintenance of a community mental health program include the following: thoroughly investigate as many aspects of the community as possible, with particular emphasis on the various citizen groups necessary for cooperation; clarify whether the goals correspond with those of the community; assess the actual and potential sources of conflict between different groups to allow for preventive mediation; try to effect and coordinate existing power groups; inform and attempt to involve community members with their own goals; endeavor to anticipate certain problem areas; and set realistic goals in order not to frustrate the community and oneself (25). Once these issues have been heeded, one can focus on the most pressing and crucial needs. This effort would primarily involve bridging gaps in services, particularly after high-risk groups have been identified. It makes sense to start in areas most deprived in terms of treatment settings, housing, and vocational and recreational facilities. Although a number of well-thought-out programs (18, 72) have been established, there is no guarantee for success, as the variables are too numerous to control. Thus a number of settings did not survive the first few years because their white, middle-class staff was just not acceptable to a largely poor and black population at the height of the black civil rights' movement in the mid-sixties.

After all has been planned and implemented how does one know whether one has accomplished what one intended? One could rely on anecdotal evidence, but in the age of accountability, peer review, and cost effectiveness, this evidence might not be impressive enough. Politically oriented and/or motivated program evaluations have been suggested (81) and have run justifiably I think (owing to contentious parameters of efficacy and success) into a great deal of professional opposition. Unfortunately, as Cowan pointed out in a recent review of evaluation and research of community services, our obsession with precise and objective data is unlikely to be satisfied in this field. He stated that "realities of the community context militate against good program evaluation research. Many limiting factors in such research stem from a clash in values between those who must deliver and those who must evaluate community services." Cowan and Klerman list some of the reasons for this difficulty in evaluation: the issues involved are of extraordinary complexity and in a constant state of flux. Furthermore, the service orientation along with a susceptibility to day-to-day pressures present realistically serious obstacles to a clean laboratory style research (27, 77). In another study, Hedley and Tardiff stress that it is impossible to evaluate in these settings the effectiveness of any single treatment modality, because usually several forms are offered concommitantly (61). This author came to similar conclusions in a clinical setting a few years ago and observed that judgment about the effectiveness of community-based programs will have to come slowly in an accumulative fashion from a variety of experiences and studies (27, 120).

Impact on Mental Health Care Delivery

The implementation of de-institutionalization policies brought with it a massive shift of patients from the state mental hospitals to facilities in the community. Chronic schizophrenics formed the largest group in this population (78). These patients could not just blend into the surrounding society at large and, thus, a comprehensive network of cooperating and coordinated facilities was needed to accommodate them (35). As this author pointed out in a previous study, the issue of integrative services becomes a paramount one with a population replete with multiple medical, social, and legal problems (120).

Ideally these facilities should include (aside from the local community mental health centers) a variety of settings that would also be responsive to the medical, housing, vocational, and recreational needs of the target population. Patients need to have unencumbered access to inpatient and outpatient medical services, whether utilizing individual physicians, private clinics, or public facilities.

Housing is a particularly crucial issue. In many instances the patient does not have a family to go back to, or it is not advisable for him/her to do so for his/her own sake. Frequently the family does not want the patient back after repeated and/or prolonged hospitalizations (120). Therefore halfway houses and other special residential facilities, whether privately owned or government subsidized initially, with varying degrees of professional supervision, represent one of the most important aspects of aftercare (3, 28, 132, 142). For the more severely disturbed patients, boarding houses with a live-in landlord who can provide meals and supervise medication-taking are preferable. A recent study by Bergman et al. indicated that demented elderly patients do best with their families and not just with an older spouse.

The extra help to these families from the social services seems to be well worth its cost (13). Sheltered workshops for vocational evaluation, retraining, and at times lifelong employment are a must. Many of the discharged patients are unable to function on their previous levels at work, and others have been on welfare for years. In such a new setting many will get a chance to become gainfully employed again. Besides, through the process of socialization and attention getting, further positive effects on patient morale are achieved. Experience in a variety of metropolitan areas indicates that these workshops play a pivotal role in the rehabilitation of chronic patients (120, 121, 126).

Because of the patient's long-term inhospital treatment and the residual effects of the illness, subsequent social isolation in this population is rampant. Therefore, a somewhat structured social and recreational programming is indispensable. Usually one or more professional or volunteer facilitators will oversee the activities in an ex-patient club (15, 119, 120) or sports facility, where discussion groups, dances, games, and a variety of sports can take place. Most of these shelter-care organizations strive toward autonomy in financial and policy matters. Many of them emphasize an intensive but transitional involvement with their clients, aiming eventually at a more independent integration within society (58).

There are certain individual patients or groups requiring specific services. Patients who are physically invalid or who are uncooperative and some children do benefit from a home visit (58) by a social worker or a public health nurse, as British and Canadian experience has shown (52, 120). Furthermore, children, adolescents, the aged, alcoholics, and drug addicts, just to mention some of the larger groups, require special facilities with particular expertise. Services for the repeating and long-term substance users necessitate the establishment of a one-stop clinic, where a team approach offers a comprehensive psychosocial, medical, vocational, and recreational counseling and management (120).

The complexity of aftercare demands a continuity of care that cannot be achieved without each patient having a mental health professional to coordinate his/her management (57). According to Holder, "The most desirable way to achieve accountability for the client is to have an agent of the system who represents the client and negotiates the services and supports the client's needs" (66). This approach cuts down on duplication of services, reduces the chances of rehospitalization, and adds immensely to the patient's sense of belonging and feeling that someone does care. The tendency of these patients to be difficult, to make little headway in therapy, to fail to keep appointments, and to make often enormous demands on the therapist does affect the latter's morale and is detrimental to the notion of continuity of care. Owing to these factors, the chronic patients are among the most unwanted in our field (23, 75).

Coordination is equally essential on a community or metropolitan level (5). The larger the population and support services involved, the more difficult it is to know what happens where, how, and why. The individual client or agency will miss opportunities if no proper integration of all available information occurs. Large cities and scattered rural communities would therefore greatly benefit from a "super agency," a service for services, such as developed in Toronto (120) and a few other cities. In the Toronto model, Community Resources Consultants was "designed to integrate existing services, mediate between the referring facility and 'receptor' facilities, follow-up on patient placements, to gather information as to the adequacy and/or appropriateness of the facilities, stimulate the development of new facilities as gaps in the service network are identified, and maintain a constant evaluative surveillance of the entire program" (46).

How did the proliferation of community-based mental health services affect patient treatment and aftercare? Copious research indicates a dramatic exodus of patients from mental hospitals to outpatient facilities. Gruenberg found in 1966 a 50 percent decrease in bed occupancy in mental hospitals over the previous decade (55). Bassuk and Gerson found a 65 percent reduction in the census of resident patients in mental hospitals in the United States between 1955 and 1975. Concomitantly they registered more than a doubling of outpatient contacts (11). Smith et al. have documented in a midwestern region that the mean length of stay of patients hospitalized for the first time dropped from 81 to 33 days, within the five years preceding 1970 (129).

The reduction of the chronic population in mental hospitals was comparably impressive in other countries. Between 1960 and 1970, their numbers diminished by 40 percent in Ontario (46). In the same period, the British were able to eliminate 24,000 beds in the mental hospitals, and this decline in the number of beds still continues (37). Further studies carried out in Finland, Germany, Norway, and England corroborated this trend (1, 94, 100, 128).

More specifically, the efficacy, feasibility, safety, and cost effectiveness of the combined psychotropic and psychosocial treatments outside institutions have been tested. A study by Zwerling and Wilder showed that up to 80 percent of patients destined for inpatient care could be successfully managed in a day-treatment setting (145). Sainsbury in Britain documented a lower readmission rate where adequate community facilities were available (118). Windle and Scully in a study of sixteen states, pointed out a decrease in state hospital admissions in areas where community mental health centers were located (139). Pasamanick et al. have demonstrated home treatment by nurses to represent a viable alternative to hospitalization (102). In addition, various studies have documented the feasibility and efficacy of short, intensive hospitalization for the acutely ill, including psychotic patients (47, 51, 63, 64). Klerman stated that appropriate community care reduced the number of chronic patients in institutions by about 60 percent (78). The main beneficiaries of this trend toward outpatient care have been the poor (125) and young adults. On the other hand, the elderly, children, alcoholics, and drug addicts have not been well looked after (8).

Specific Issues

The models from which most of the community-based programs are derived have been thought of in terms of their effect on the white adult residents in need in urban areas. Because of these conceptual origins, large segments of the population have been inadequately looked after and neglected.

One such group has been the large rural population. The magnitude of the problem can be gauged by the fact that in the United States alone, the rural population comprises about fifty million people. Rural counties constitute the major part of the nation's land area (24). Many of the problems connected with the delivery of mental health services in rural areas have to do with their sheer size. A large portion of their budgets has to be spent on transportation and communication (10). Therefore mental health professionals will frequently have less time for direct treatment. That fact alone makes them more vulnerable in comparison with their urban colleagues, in terms of productivity. In addition, because of the paucity of manpower, the mental health professional has to be a generalist rather than a specialist, at a time when funding has been contingent on the provision of specialized services (24). Anonymity and confidentiality are much more difficult to achieve in many small communities, and resistance to change is stronger. Rural mental health workers frequently suffer from professional isolation, and yet feel penalized by continuing education requirements, which for them are much more difficult to obtain. The result is a very high staff turnover rate in many of the affected areas. On the positive side, usually a strong sense of community prevails among the population, and there is a better opportunity for the therapist to have firsthand observations of patients. This attitude can lead to more direct and humane decisions in treatment (92).

The recommendations of the Report of the President's Commission on Mental Health (5) should provide a much-needed impetus to improve the situation in rural areas in the long run. Other until recently neglected segments of the population likely to benefit from the Commission's work are children, adolescents, the elderly, alcoholics, drug addicts, the poor, and minorities, who might have been socially, culturally, and linguistically too disadvantaged to utilize even the available services.

Industry and institutions for higher education in North America have generally been less successful rehabilitating their members who became chronically mentally ill than those in some other countries (74, 121). The school system and the armed forces have generally a better record to show.

Not all the brunt in the process of de-institutionalization has been born by the patients or the community alone. Mental health professionals, carrying out the policies in the "front line," have had serious morale and identity problems. In a thorough study Pines and Maslach have eloquently described "staff burnout" in mental health settings (106). The workers in these facilities felt overwhelmed and demoralized by the high-intensity, crisis-oriented approach, with few visible or acknowledged rewards. They tended to fend for themselves by intellectualization, distancing, and detachment. These researchers concluded, as does this author (120) that the function of the staff meeting should be primarily to socialize informally, to give each other support, to discuss problem patients, to offer a real opportunity to express feelings, and to have input into some control over their own work routines. The goal setting for and by each individual therapist should be realistic, to avoid the frustration accompanying the feeling that one is never going to "catch up" with ever escalating demands. Many professionals suffer in community settings from an "identity diffusion" and an overextension of their commitments and roles (11, 60, 89). Levinson, Klerman, Lowy, and others have pointed out the risks involved in assuming responsibilities in mental health facilities for which one's training has not adequately prepared the provider (78, 87, 89). This author could not agree more with a discussant at a recent conference, who stated that mental health professionals "were lost as we got into management, systems evaluation, cost-benefit analysis, community responsiveness, third-party payers, and accreditation. It is very far afield from our clinical training" (108). Unless the potentially positive aspects and the rewards in this difficult area are going to be given proper recognition by the institutional leadership, this process of attrition will continue (88). Therefore, it is recommended that more emphasis in the professional training at the under- and postgraduate level should be put on preparation for community- and team-oriented mental health care delivery (78, 87, 89, 141).

One of the cornerstones of successful community follow-up is the free accessibility of the health care delivery system. This accessibility was accomplished a generation ago through the National Health Service in Britain, over a decade ago in Canada, and partially in the United States in the form of Medicare and Medicaid. The public insurance systems for the first time in the two former countries acknowledged the equality of physical and mental illness in terms of comprehensive coverage. Fears have persisted, though, that in a universal coverage people would be "overtreated" owing to a tendency to self-exploration and self-actualization. The supposed "incurability" of most emotional disorders added a further argument in this direction (127). However, data from provincial medical care insurance programs in Canada indicated that the proportion of psychiatric payments out of the total medical ones amounted to 1.4

percent to 5.4 percent only (109). Furthermore, mental health center data from Kentucky showed that 87% of the patients were seen for ten or less visits (39). Even county and state mental hospitals had an average stay of less than thirty days (39). A study by Jameson et al. revealed, moreover, that money spent on outpatient psychotherapy may be offset by the lower utilization of medical-surgical services by the same people (69). It seems that the most powerful force for or against the financing of mental health programs has been the vocal strength and lobbying power of a citizen's alliance and of a professional or a political pressure group, short of the influence of a presidential spouse.

Critical Appraisal

The achievements of the community mental health movement with its emphasis on de-institutionalization cannot be ignored. Both acutely ill and chronic patients spend much less time in institutions, which, in themselves, have become more attuned to their residents' needs. Mental health professionals, administrators, and politicians became more optimistic about treatment prospects, and as a result large sums of money have been invested in alternate care and rehabilitation facilities in the community. However, the policy of early discharge of acute patients and the community placement of long-stay hospital patients represented primarily administrative changes, which concealed a considerable amount of real social disability (129). Klerman observed that the chronic mentally ill are "better but not well." Their limited ability to lead independent social lives evokes multiple problems for public welfare, urban zoning, health care agencies, and legal institutions (78). Increasing concern has been expressed regarding the social and community costs involved and the burdens imposed on the psychiatric patients in an environment they cannot cope with (6, 29). Much of the positive assessment of our achievements has been simplistic, primarily quantitative, and embellished by self-fulfilling prophecies.

The initiation of many community-based programs and their funding has been a political act with inadequate prior research (77). Often the popularity of the program has been the rationale for its funding

(134). Health policies have been formulated primarily on the basis of beliefs and attitudes, uncritically linking cause-and-effect issues (6). Some of these assumptions seem to have taken on the form of myths, reflecting more the hopes and expectations of the community mental health movement than the uncomfortable realities (75). Furthermore, as Panzetta pointed out, the community mental health movement has glorified the concept of community, without full understanding. Instead of being characterized by an implicit bond with common values, care for each other, mutual dependence, and respect, our real communities have formal and explicit bonds. People's relationships are affected by formulated guidelines, rules, and regulations. Caring and dependence on another for survival rarely exist (101). This lack of adequate conceptualization has serious negative implications for the proper implementation of community programs for the chronic cases of mental illness.

By keeping the patient *out* of the hospital, it was assumed that he/she would be kept *in* the community (75). However, many of the former patients were transients in any given location (40) or had lost their identification with that community during the course of their long hospitalization. Thus, the belief in the advantages of reintegration has been devoid of any serious analysis of what constitutes a relevant community.

In addition, the *community* was not ready for the task assigned to it. While some of the earlier biases toward the mentally ill had lessened, enough prejudice survived to hamper seriously the settling of ex-patients in "normal" neighborhoods. Carstairs and Wing stated over a generation ago that the "social isolation of mental hospital patients is due in part to the way in which they are perceived by the general public" (20), and this phenomenon is still true today. Our society uses subtle ways of keeping the mental patients out of a "desirable" neighborhood by zoning restrictions, city ordinances, and police interventions (7, 42). These efforts tend to increase further their concentration in poorer, less cohesive and disorganized areas of the cities. Social rejection of the mentally disordered, which has been amply documented (7, 22, 70, 75, 104, 115, 123, 124, 135, 138), often led to the replacement of the mental hospital by an even more miserable, isolated, dehumanizing, and frightening existence in the worst ghetto areas of inner cities (9, 82, 97, 143).

Many former chronic patients live in substandard, overcrowded, dirty, and unsafe houses and have minimal activities and little interaction with the surrounding people. These individuals are at the mercy of their landlords, the bureaucrats in the welfare agencies, and harassing neighbors. Reich and Siegal give a vivid description of the real conditions in such areas: "an even more oppressive, appalling state of affairs is unfolding, as rooming houses, foster homes, nursing homes, and run-down hotels take the place of former back wards. Here the discharged patients are frequently clustered—unsupervised, unmedicated, uncared for, frequently the prey of unscrupulous and criminal elements" (111). Others are placed in nursing homes, convalescent facilities, and homes for the aged, where they receive inferior, or no treatment, and are as much socially isolated as in the old asylums. This process has been justifiably labeled by the Department of Health, Education and Welfare as "reinstitutionalization" (11). Kramer noted that while the transfer of large numbers of elderly mental patients from the public hospitals to nursing homes has improved dramatically the de-institutionalization statistics, it is doubtful whether such a community transfer contributes to the patient's quality of life and longevity (80).

The mass movement of patients from the state hospitals was as a rule not accompanied by a concomitant expansion of community services. Many of the discharged patients were lost in their new environment and because of their often bizarre behavior became neighborhood nuisances and objects of fear. Numerous patients ended up in prisons (112), where conditions were likely to be worse than in most mental hospitals. Rehabilitation and social integration was almost nonexistent for many of them (99). Even the Department of Health and Social Security in Britain, previously a vigorous advocate of de-institutionalization, recently sounded a warning: "those who work in the health and social services field have to recognize that families and relatives, and indeed the public at large cannot be expected to tolerate under the name of community care the discharge of chronic patients without adequate arrangements being made for aftercare and who perhaps spent their days wandering the streets or become an unbearable burden on the lives of their relatives . . . " (36). Administrators and policy planners did not anticipate the pressures and stress to which patients and their families became exposed. Such a forced interaction had detrimental effects on all involved.

Little was done to determine if indeed the community cared and if its support systems were adequate. In this way, the "open-door" policy of yesterday has evolved into the "revolving-door" approach of today (115). Therefore it is not surprising that the readmission rates in Ontario rose by 300 percent in the decade preceding 1970 (46).

Many reliable studies from different geographic regions tend to underline the illusory nature of the de-institutionalization statistics. According to Bassuk and Gerson, in 1972 64 percent of all admissions to mental hospitals were readmissions. Furthermore, half of the re-leased patients were readmitted within one year (11). Similar results were observed by Anthony, Gunderson, Smith, and others (4, 5, 6, 76, 93, 129). Moreover, it became clear that reintegration into society at large, even under optimal conditions, was more likely to be successful with acute patients than with those who had long histories of (often repeated) hospitalizations (55).

Aside from the human and ethical issues involved, the expected fiscal savings from a community-based program played a major role in the push for de-institutionalization. This hope has not materialized because effective extramural care requires very large expenditures. Significant numbers of patients living outside the hospital need a gamut of welfare, medical, housing, legal, vocational, and recreational services, and it is very doubtful whether any financial advantages accrue in this approach (11, 75, 82, 143). Instead, as Chu and Trotter observed, because of a new ideology and availability, a different (until now unserviced) clientele has been attracted to swell the ranks of the beneficiaries (23).

In summary, the trend toward the de-institutionalization of the mentally ill was a much-needed, well-intended, but ill-researched endeavor. Much hope and enthusiasm dissipated under the impact of harsh realities and insight gained over the past generation. A backlash among politicians and mental health professionals alike threatens many positive achievements unless the expectations can be adjusted to the art of the possible.

Future Trends and Recommendations

A good indication as to the direction in which community mental health services are likely to develop in the future is contained in the recent Report of the President's Commission on Mental Health (5). It acknowledges the need for increased federal funding. This need has been advocated by a number of reputable experts for a while (11, 16, 17, 83), should the programs maintain and expand their scope. For the first time there is a tacit acceptance of the fact that no amount of effort at the present level of our knowledge will eradicate all chronic mental illness. In the light of this understanding greater emphasis will be placed on the management of the chronically ill. Funding priority will be given to populations who have special needs and who live in underserved areas.

Universal and comprehensive health insurance systems have been found to be expensive by governments; they seem cumbersome with a tendency to foster bureaucracy in the eyes of some mental health professionals and many patients in various countries. Nevertheless, this framework seems to have represented the lesser evil for the President's Commission. In such a plan the reimbursement would go to a facility, rather than to an individual (5). This system is designed to foster a multidisciplinary approach, within the guidelines of minimal training and accreditation criteria. There is no doubt that it is expected at the same time to keep health care delivery costs within manageable limits. (It seems, however, that again wishful thinking and ideology have been substituted for thorough research.)

As demand has far outstripped available personnel, an emphasis will have to be placed on early and realistic training of mental health professionals. Moreover, proper remuneration and considerably more attention will have to be given to the working milieu of the community worker with all its problems to avoid a high turnover rate and demoralization. Clinical evidence and numerous well-designed research studies have proved beyond reasonable doubt the inversely reciprocal relationship between the availability of aftercare and read-mission rates. Hogarthy, Gruenberg, Kirk, and others have shown that the lowest degree of rehospitalization was associated with the combination of pharmaco- and psychosocial therapies utilized by the patient (19, 43, 44, 55, 62, 65, 76, 84). In order to achieve maximal effects for the patient at an acceptable cost, it is crucial that the community services be better integrated and coordinated (16).

Communities should develop viable alternatives *before* pressuring for the closure of mental hospitals so that patients will not have to pay for sociopolitical lip sevice by "jumping from the fire into the frying pan." As the number of the emotionally ill requiring outpatient treatment is considerable, coopcration with othcr psychiatric facilities, including mental hospitals and primary care providers is essential (17, 110).

Even an increased allocation of funds will necessitate setting careful priorities for future expansion of services. Establishing priorities is imperative to prevent getting bogged down in an attempt to "bite off more than we can chew." By implication, we cannot try to tackle the problems of schizophrenia, alcoholism, drug addiction, child and geriatric psychiatry, poverty, and minorities *all* at once. Judicious decisions will have to be made, primarily taking into account available evidence, rather than social or political expediency. Consequently, primary preventive programs should not be at the top of the list, aside from a few specific instances (83).

Furthermore, we shall have to acknowledge that while comprehensive aftercare services are highly desirable, they are often not feasible in reality. Thus the availability of less inclusive facilities can compensate for their incompleteness. This benefit is particularly true if a specific service is to be tested out or if it is seen as a base-line operation to be expanded, if and when more experience and finances become handy (5, 30, 68, 120). This notion is implied in President Jimmy Carter's Commission on Mental Health, which talks about "Community Mental Health *Systems*"— stressing the fact that coordination is more essential in practice than comprehensiveness (5).

Needs of the patients and of their families should be heeded, and more attention will have to be payed to their views. It is one thing to agree with the "motherhood" statement that old-fashioned, large mental institutions are detrimental to their residents, but should we ignore at the same time the patient's preferences? It is this author's contention that most chronic patients deserve the right to be truly consulted regarding their post-acute management. There is strong accumulating evidence to suggest, as the spokesman of the National Schizophrenia Fellowship (98) pointed out, that for many patients small or medium-sized asylums in the old sense, but of more recent orientation, are preferable to the isolation, degradation, and anomie in their nonexistent community (11, 115).

In fact the readmission of some psychiatric patients is necessary for short periods during an exacerbation, just as it is at times necessary to admit a decompensated cardiac patient. At times, the need may be there on behalf of the chronic patient to seek refuge in an asylum, as a way to deal with the intolerance his/her family or community has exhibited toward him/her or vice versa (50).

As long as public misunderstanding and fear of mental disorder will persist, the care of the long-term psychiatrically ill in society at large will be hampered. Despite significant improvement over the past quarter of a century, much still needs changing. There is no sure way to end discriminatory feelings and practices. The President's Commission recommended more research into people's attitudes toward mental illness in order to develop more successful educational programs. The public media in the United States will receive more relevant information through a coordinated resources center to be established by private mental health organizations (5).

The management of chronic patients is the cornerstone of all community-based programs in the field of mental health. A society will be judged not only upon its statements and beliefs but also upon its accomplishments. For us on this continent, there is no reason at this time to feel either jubilant or resigned. Although our goals in the past were overly ambitious and optimistic, with a lot more foresight, humility, and flexibility we still have the foundation of the potentially best mental health system anywhere.

References

1. Achte, K. A., & Apo, M. Schizophrenic patients in 1950–1951 and 1956–1959: A comparative study. *Psychiatric Quarterly* 41: 422–441, 1967.

2. Alexander, F. G., & Selesnick, S. T. *The History of Psychiatry*. New York: The New American Library, A Mentor Book, 1966.

3. Anstee, B. H. An alternative to group homes. *British Journal of Psychiatry* 132: 356–360, 1978.

4. Anthony, W. A., Buell, G. J., Sharratt, S., & Althoff, M. E. Efficacy of psychiatric rehabilitation. *Psychological Bulletin* 78: 447–456, 1972.

5. Armstrong, B. The report of the president's commission on mental health: A summary of recommendations. *Hospital and Community Psychiatry* 29: 7, 468–474, 1978.

6. Arnhoff, F. N. Social consequences of policy toward mental illness. *Science* 188: 1277–1281, 1975.

7. Aviram, U., & Segal, S. P. Exclusion of the mentally ill. *Archives of General Psychiatry* 29: 126–131, 1973.

8. Babigian, H. M. The impact of community mental health centers on the utilization of services. *Archives of General Psychiatry* 34: 385–394, 1977.

9. Bachrach, L. L. A note on some recent studies of released mental hospital patients in the community. *American Journal of Psychiatry* 133: 1, 73–75, 1976.

10. Bachrach, L. L. De-institutionalization of mental health services in rural areas. *Hospital and Community Psychiatry* 28: 9, 669–672, 1977.

11. Bassuk, E. L., & Gerson, S. De-institutionalization and mental health services. *Scientific American* 238: 2, 46–53, 1978.

12. Belknap, I. *Human Problems of a State Mental Hospital*. New York: McGraw-Hill, 1956.

13. Bergmann, K., Foster, E. M., Justice, A. W., & Matthews, V. Management of the demented elderly patient in the community. *British Journal Psychiatry* 132: 441–449, 1978.

14. Bettelheim, B., & Sylvester, E. A therapeutic milieu. *American Journal of Orthopsychiatry* 18: 191–206, 1948.

15. Bierer, J. England's therapeutic social clubs. *Mental Hospital* 13: 203–207, 1962.

16. Borus, J. F., Janowitch, L. A., Kiefer, F., Morrill, R. G., Reich, L., Simone, E., & Towle, L. The coordination of mental health services at the neighbourhood level. *American Journal of Psychiatry* 132: 11, 1177–1181, 1975.

17. Borus, J. F. Issues critical to the survival of community mental health. *American Journal of Psychiatry* 135: 9, 1029–1035, 1978.

18. Brickman, H. R. Organization of a community mental health program in a metropolis. In G. Caplan (ed.), *American Handbook of Psychiatry*, Volume 2. New York: Basic Books, 1974, pp. 662–672.

19. Byers, E. S., Cohen, S., & Harshbarger, D. D. Impact of aftercare services on recidivism of mental hospital patients. *Community Mental Health Journal* 14: 26–34, 1978.

20. Carstairs, G. M., & Wing, J. K. Attitudes of the general public to mental illness. *British Medical Journal* 2: 594–597, 1958.

21. Caudill, W. *The Psychiatric Hospital as a Small Society*. Cambridge, Mass.: Harvard University Press, 1958.

22. Chase, J. Where have all the patients gone? *Human Behavior* 14–21, October 1973.

23. Chu, F., & Trotter, S. *The Madness Establishment*. Grossman, 1974.

24. Clayton, T. Issues in the delivery of rural mental health services. *Hospital and Community Psychiatry* 28: 9, 673–676, 1977.

25. Cohen, R. E. Community organizational aspects of establishing and maintaining a local program. In G. Caplan (ed.), *American Handbook of Psychiatry*, Volume 2. New York: Basic Books, 1974, pp. 649–661.

26. Conolly, J. *The Treatment of the Insane without Mechanical Restraints*. London: Smith, Elder and Company, 1856.

27. Cowen, E. L. Some problems in community program evaluation research. *Journal of Consulting and Clinical Psychology* 46: 792–805, 1978.

28. Craft, M., & Wilkins, R. Residential needs in hospital and the community for mentally handicapped people. *British Journal Psychiatry* 132: 450–454, 1978.

29. Crane, G. E. Two decades of psychopharmacology and community mental health: Old and new problems of the schizophrenic patient. *Transactions of the New York Academy of Sciences* 36: 644–656, 1974.

30. Crichton, A. Community health centers: Health care organization of the future? Information Canada, Department of Health and Welfare, Canada. 1973, pp. 19-1–19-2.

31. Davis, E. B. The role of the psychiatrist in "The chronic patient": Perspectives from the 29th Institute on hospital and community psychiatry. *Hospital and Community Psychiatry* 29: 1, 33, 1978.

32. Davis, J. E. The rights of chronic patients. *Hospital and Community Psychiatry* 29: 1, 39, 1978.

33. David, J. M. Overview: Maintenance therapy in psychiatry: I, Schizophrenia. *American Journal of Psychiatry* 132: 1237–1295, 1975.

34. Davis, J. M., & Cole, J. O. Antipsychotic drugs. In A. M. Freedman, H. I. Kaplan, & B. J. Sadock (eds।)., *Comprehensive Textbook of Psychiatry*, Volume 2. Baltimore: The Williams and Wilkins Company, 1975, p. 1921.

35. Demone, H. W., Jr. Human services at state and local levels: The integration of mental health. In G. Caplan (ed.), *American Handbook of Psychiatry*, Volume 2. New York: Basic Books, 1974, pp. 557–592.

36. Department of Health and Social Security. *Better Services for the Mentally Ill*. Cmnd 6233. London: Her Majesty's Stationery Office, 1975.

37. Department of Health and Social Security. Psychiatric hospitals and units in England. In-patient statistics from the mental health enquiry for the

year 1973. *Statistical and Research Report Services* 12. London: Her Majesty's Stationery Office, 1976.

38. Deutsch, D. *The Mentally Ill in America*. Garden City, N.Y.: Doubleday, Doran and Company, 1937.

39. Draft Report. The financing, utilization and quality of mental health care in the United States. Rockville, Md: National Institute of Mental Health Office of Program Development and Analysis, April 1976.

40. Dunham, E. *Community and Schizophrenia*. Detroit: Wayne State University Press, 1965.

41. Ellenberger, H. Zoological garden and mental hospital. *Canadian Psychiatric Association Journal* 5: 136–149, 1960.

42. Elpers, J. R. Legal constraints in providing community care. *Hospital and Community Psychiatry* 29: 1, 37, 1978.

43. Fairweather, G. E., Sanders, D. H., Cressler, D. L., & Maynard, H. *Community Life for the Mentally Ill*. Chicago: Aldine Publication Company, 1969.

44. Fakhruddin, A. K. M., Manjooran, A., Nair, N. P. V., et al. A five year outcome of discharged chronic psychiatric patients. *Canadian Psychiatric Association Journal* 17: 433–435, 1972.

45. Fischer-Homberger, E. Germany and Austria. In J. C. Howells (ed.), *World History of Psychiatry*. New York: Brunner and Mazel, 1975, pp. 273–275.

46. Fisher, L., & Freeman, S. J. J. Community Resources Consultants: An experimental approach to aftercare. *Canada's Mental Health* 24: 1, 33–36, 1976.

47. Glick, I. D., Hargreaves, W. A., Drues, J., & Schostak, J. A. Short versus long hospitalization: A prospective controlled study IV. One year follow-up results for schizophrenic patients. *American Journal of Psychiatry* 133: 509–514, 1976.

48. Goffman, E. The moral career of mental patients. *Psychiatry* 22: 123–142, 1959.

49. Goffman, E. *Asylums*. New York: Doubleday, 1961.

50. Green, R. S., & Rabiner, D. J. Making rehospitalization part of the plan. In The chronic patient: Perspectives from the 29th Institute on hospital and community psychiatry. *Hospital and Community Psychiatry* 29: 1, 36–37, 1978.

51. Greenblatt, M., Solomon, M., Evans, A. S., & Brooks, G. W., eds. Drugs and social therapy in chronic schizophrenia. Springfield, Ill.: Charles C. Thomas Publication, 1965.

52. Greene, J. Discharge and be damned. *The Royal Society of Health Journal* 93: 3, 104–107, 1978.

53. Griesinger, W. *Die Pathologie und Therapie der psychischen Krankheiten.* Stuttgart: Adolph Krabbe, 1845, pp. 347–351.

54. Grob, G. N. *Mental Institutions in America: Social Policy to 1895.* New York: Free Press, 1973.

55. Gruenberg, E. M., ed. Evaluating the effectiveness of community mental health services. *Millbank Memorial Fund Quarterly* 44, pt. 2, 1966.

56. Gunderson, J. Special report: Schizophrenia, 1974. *Schizophrenia Bulletin* 16–54, Summer 1974.

57. Gurevitz, H. Caring for chronic patients: Some cautions and concerns. *Hospital and Community Psychiatry* 29: 1, 42–43, 1978.

58. Hansell, N. The elements of a local service program. In G. Caplan (ed.), *American Handbook of Psychiatry,* Volume 2. New York: Basic Books, 1974, pp. 627–648.

59. [Hastings, J. E. F.]. Report of the community health centre project of the conference of health ministers. *Canadian Medical Association Journal* 107: 361–380, 1972.

60. Hauser, W. Process problems in community psychiatry. *American Journal of Psychiatry* 126: 112–116, 1969.

61. Hedley, R. A., Graham, B. J., Cooper, M., Macurdy, E. A., & Tardiff, K. J. Community mental health teams: An observational study. *Social Science and Medicine* 12: 265–270, 1978.

62. Herjanic, M., Stewart, D., & Hales, R. C. The chronic patient in the community. *Canadian Psychiatric Association Journal* 13: 231–235, 1968.

63. Herz, M. I., Endicott, J., Spitzer, R. L., & Mesnikoff, A. Day versus inpatient hospitalization: A controlled study. *American Journal of Psychiatry* 127: 1371–1382, 1971.

64. Herz, M. I., Endicott, J., & Spitzer, R. L. Brief hospitalization of patients with families: Initial results. *American Journal of Psychiatry* 132: 413–418, 1975.

65. Hogarty, G. E., Goldberg, S. C., & The Collaborative Study Group. Drug and sociotherapy in the aftercare of schizophrenic patients: One year relapse rates. *Archives of General Psychiatry* 28: 1, 54–64, 1973.

66. Holder, H. D. Building accountability into the service system. *Hospital and Community Psychiatry* 29: 1, 38–39, 1978.

67. Howells, J. G., & Osborn, M. L. Great Britain. In J. G. Howells (ed.), *World History of Psychiatry.* New York: Brunner and Mazel, 1975, pp. 192–206.

68. Hume, P. B. Principles of community mental health practice. In G. Caplan (ed.), *American Handbook of Psychiatry,* Volume 2. New York: Basic Books, 1974, pp. 615–626.

69. Jameson, J., Shuman, L. J., & Young, W. E. The effects of outpatient

psychiatric utilization on the costs of providing third-party coverage. *Medical Care* 16: 5, 383–399, 1978.

70. Joint Commission on Mental Illness and Mental Health. *Action for Mental Health*. New York: Basic Books, 1961.

71. Jones, M. *The Therapeutic Community*. New York: Basic Books, 1953.

72. Kellam, S. G., & Schiff, S. K. The Woodlawn mental health center: A community mental health center model. *Social Services Review* 40: 3, 255–263, 1966.

73. Kennedy, J. F. Message from the President of the United States relative to mental illness and mental retardation. House of Representatives document no. 58, 88th Congress, 1st session. February 5, 1963. Washington, D.C.: United States Government Printing Office, 1963.

74. Kiev, A. *Psychiatry in the Communist World*. New York: Science House, 1968, pp. 23–25.

75. Kirk, S. A., & Therrien, M. E. Community mental health myths and the fate of former hospitalized patients. *Psychiatry* 38: 209–217, 1975.

76. Kirk, S. A. Effectiveness of community services for discharged mental hospital patients. *American Journal of Orthopsychiatry* 46: 4, 646–659, 1976.

77. Klerman, G. Current evaluation research on mental health services. *American Journal of Psychiatry* 131: 7, 783–787, 1974.

78. Klerman, G. L. Better but not well: Social and ethical issues in the de-institutionalization of the mentally ill. *Schizophrenia Bulletin* 3: 4, 617–631, 1977.

79. Kraepelin, E. *Hundert Jahre Psychiatrie*. Berlin: Julius Springer, Berlin, 1918, pp. 106–108.

80. Kramer, M. Applications of mental health statistics: Uses in mental health programs of statistics derived from psychiatric services and selected vital and morbidity records. Geneva, Switzerland. World Health Organization, 1969. In G. L. Klerman, Better but not well: Social and ethical issues in the deinstitutionalization of the mentally ill. *Schizophrenia Bulletin* 3: 4, 617–631, 1977.

81. Krause, M. S., & Howard, K. I. Program evaluation in the public interest: A new research methodology. *Community Mental Health Journal* 12: 3, 291–300, 1976.

82. Lamb, H. R., & Goerzel, V. Discharged mental patients—are they really in the community? *Archives of General Psychiatry* 24: 29–34, 1971.

83. Lamb, H. R., & Zusman, J. Primary prevention in perspective. *American Journal of Psychiatry* 136: 1, 12–17, 1979.

84. Lafave, H. G., Stewart, A., & Grunberg, F. Community care of the

mentally ill: Implementation of the Saskatchewan plan. *Community Mental Health Journal* 4: 37–45, 1968.

85. Lehmann, H. E. Psychopharmacological treatment of schizophrenia. *Schizophrenia Bulletin* 1: 13, 27–45, 1975.

86. Levenson, A. I. A review of the federal community mental health centers program. In G. Caplan (ed.), *American Handbook of Psychiatry*, Volume 2. New York: Basic Books, 1974, pp. 593–604.

87. Levinson, D. J., & Klerman, G. L. The clinician executive. *Psychiatry* 30: 4, 3–15, 1967.

88. Lipp, M. R. What's in it for the therapist? In The chronic patient: Perspectives from the 29th Institute on hospital and community psychiatry. *Hospital and Community Psychiatry* 29: 1, 40–41, 1978.

89. Lowy, F. H. The impact of community psychiatry on psychiatric teaching. In J. Divic, & M. Dinoff (eds.), *Aspects of Community Psychiatry: Review and Preview*. University, Ala.: The University of Alabama Press, 1978, pp. 93–101.

90. Macht, L. B. Community psychiatry. In A. M. Nichols (ed.), *The Harvard Guide to Modern Psychiatry*. Cambridge, Mass.: Harvard University Press, 1978, p. 628.

91. Margetts, E. L. Canada. *World History of Psychiatry*. New York: Brunner and Mazel, 1975, pp. 417–431.

92. Mazer, M. *People and Predicaments*. Cambridge, Mass.: Harvard University Press, 1976, p. 215.

93. *Mental Health of East London in 1966*. London: Psychiatric Rehabilitation Association, 1968.

94. Meyer, J. E., Simon, G., & Stille, G. Die Therapie der Schizophrenie und der endogenen Depression zwischen 1930–1960. *Archiv fuer Psychiatrie und Nervenkrankheiten vereinigt mit Zeitschrift fuer die gesamte Neurologie und Psychiatrie* 206: 165, 1964.

95. Mora, G. Italy. In J. G. Howells (ed.), *World History of Psychiatry*. New York: Brunner and Mazel, 1975, pp. 39–89.

96. Mosher, L. R. Madness and the community. *Attitude* 1: 1–10, 1972.

97. Murphy, H. B. M., Engelsman, F., & Tchenglarouche, F. The influence of foster-home care of psychiatric patients. *Archives of General Psychiatry* 33: 179–183, 1976.

98. National Schizophrenia Fellowship. *Living with schizophrenia*. Surrey, England: Surbiton, 1974.

99. Where can mental patients go? In News of the week in review. *New York Times*, February 24, 1974, p. 5.

100. Odegaard, O. Pattern of discharge from Norwegian psychiatric hospi-

tals before and after the introduction of psychotropic drugs. *American Journal of Psychiatry* 120: 772–778, 1964.

101. Panzetta, A. F. The concept of community: the short circuit of the mental health movement. *Archives of General Psychiatry* 25: 291–297, 1971.

102. Pasamanick, B., Scarpitti, F. R., & Dinitz, S. Schizophrenics in the community: An experimental study in the prevention of hospitalization. New York: Appleton-Century Crofts, 1967.

103. Pelicier, I. France. In J. G. Howells (ed.), *World History of Psychiatry*. New York: Brunner and Mazel, 1975, pp. 119–135.

104. Phillips, D. Rejection: A possible consequence of seeking help for mental disorders. *American Sociology Review* 28: 963–972, 1963.

105. Pinel, P. *A Treatise on Insanity*. Sheffield: W. Todd, 1806, pp. 48–109, 174–196.

106. Pines, A., & Maslach, C. Characteristics of staff burnout in mental health settings. *Hospital and Community Psychiatry* 29: 4, 233–237, 1978.

107. Prichard, J. C. *A Treatise on Insanity*. London: Sherwood, Gilbert and Piper, 1835, pp. 303–305.

108. Psychiatric Exodus from CMHCS. Panel examines the causes and proposes some solutions in "News and Notes." *Hospital and Community Psychiatry* 29: 6, 407–414, 1978.

109. Reed, L. S. Coverage and utilization of care for mental conditions under health insurance—various studies, 1973–1974. Washington, D.C.: American Psychiatric Association, August 1975.

110. Regier, D. A., Goldberg, I. D., & Taube, C. A. The de facto U.S. mental health services system. *Archives of General Psychiatry* 35: 685–693, 1978.

111. Reich, R., & Siegel, L. The chronically mentally ill shuffle to oblivion. *Psychiatric Annals* 3 (11): 35–55, 1974.

112. Report of the Work of the Prison Department for the Years 1961 to 1974. London: Her Majesty's Stationery Office, 1975.

113. Retterstol, N. Scandinavia and Finland. In J. G. Howells (ed.), *World History of Psychiatry*. New York: Brunner and Mazel, 1975, pp. 215–237.

114. Robbins, E., & Robbins, L. Charge to the community: Some early effects of a state hospital system's change of policy. *American Journal of Psychiatry* 131: 6, 641–645, 1974.

115. Rollin, H. R. "De-institutionalization" and the community: Fact and theory. *Psychological Medicine* 7: 181–184, 1977.

116. Rosenhan, D. L. On being sane in insane places. *Science* 179: 250–258, 1973.

117. Rothman, D. *The Discovery of the Asylum: Social Order and Disorder in the New Republic*. Boston: Little, Brown and Co., 1971.

118. Sainsbury, P. Social and community psychiatry. *American Journal of Psychiatry* 125: 9, 1226–1231, 1969.

119. Salvendy, J. T. Psychiatry in Vienna today. *Canadian Psychiatric Association Journal* 16: 2, 171–180, 1971.

120. Salvendy, J. T. A practical approach to tertiary prevention. *Israel Annals of Psychiatry* 13: 4, 364–371, 1975.

121. Salvendy, J. T. Psychiatry in the Soviet Union. *Canadian Psychiatric Association Journal* 20: 229–236, 1975.

122. Salvendy, J. T. Psychiatry in Eastern Europe: The Hungarian example. *Psychiatric Journal of the University of Ottawa* 2: 1, 43–47, 1977.

123. Sarbin, T., & Mancuso, J. Failure of a moral enterprise: Attitudes of the public toward mental illness. *Journal of Consulting and Clinical Psychology* 35: 159–173, 1970.

124. Scheff, T. *Being Mentally Ill*. Aldine, 1966.

125. Scherl, D., & English, J. Community mental health and comprehensive health service programs for the poor. *American Journal of Psychiatry* 125: 1666–1674, 1969.

126. Schulte, W., & Toelle, R. *Psychiatrie*. Berlin: Springer, Berlin, 1973, pp. 318–322.

127. Sharfstein, S. S., & Wolfe, J. C. The community mental health centers program: Expectations and realities. *Hospital and Community Psychiatry* 29: 1, 46–49, 1978.

128. Shepherd, M. Therapeutic problems with psychotropic drugs: Some epidemiological considerations. *Psychiatria, Neurologia, Neurochirurgia* 75: 503–506, 1969.

129. Smith, W. G., Krzyzanowski, M., & Heinemann, R. Impact of community mental health programs on hospitalization for mental illness. *Illinois Medical Journal* 153: 5, 359–363, 1978.

130. Stanton, A. H., & Schwartz, M. S. *The mental hospital*. New York: Basic Books, 1954.

131. Swazey, J. P. *Chlorpromazine in Psychiatry: A Study of Therapeutic Innovation*. Cambridge, Mass.: MIT Press, 1974.

132. Sylph, J. A., Eastwood, M. R., & Kedward, H. B. Long-term psychiatric care in Ontario: The homes for special care program. *Canadian Medical Association Journal* 114: 233–237, 1976.

133. The Mental Health Act. An act to amend Bill 19, 2nd Session, 31st Legislature, Ontario, 1978. Toronto: J. C. Thatcher, Queen's Printer for Ontario.

134. Toews, J. Community psychiatry: A re-examination of some concepts. *Canada's Mental Health* 25: 3–4, 1977.

135. Trotter, S., & Kuttner, B. The mentally ill: From back wards to back alleys. *Washington Post*, February 24, 1974.

136. Tuke, D. H. *The Insane in the United States and Canada*. London: H. K. Lewis, 1885, pp. 33–242.

137. U.S. Congress Community Mental Health Centers Act of 1963. Public Law 88-164, Title II. Washington, D.C.: U.S. Government Printing Office, 1963.

138. Varga, K. The placement, management and rehabilitation of the mentally ill. In G. Nyiroe (ed.), *Psychiatria*. Budapest: Medicina, 1971, pp. 204–206 (in Hungarian).

139. Windle, C., & Scully, D. Community mental health centers and the decreasing use of state mental hospitals. *Community Mental Health Journal* 12: 3, 239–243, 1976.

140. Wing, J. K. Institutionalism in mental hospitals. *British Journal of Social and Clinical Psychology* 1: 38–51, 1962.

141. Winslow, W. W. The changing role of psychiatrists in community mental health centers. *American Journal of Psychiatry* 136: 1, 24–27, 1979.

142. Winston, A., & Lieberman, H. J. Family life in community residence. *Psychiatric Quarterly* 50: 50–54, 1978.

143. Wolpert, J., Dear, M., & Drawford, R. Mental health satellite facilities in the community. Presented at the National Institute of Mental Health Center for Studies of Metropolitan Problems Seminar Series, Rockville, Md., January 1974. Quoted from G. L. Klerman, Better but not well: Social and ethical issues in the deinstitutionalization of the mentally ill. *Schizophrenia Bulletin* 3: 4, 617–631, 1977.

144. Zilboorg, G., & Henry, G. W. *A History of Medical Psychology*. New York: W. W. Norton and Co., 1969.

145. Zwerling, I., & Wilder, J. F. Day hospital treatment of psychiatric patients. *Current Psychiatric Therapy* 2: 200–210, 1962.

Clinical Role of Religion:
New Vistas or Perceptions

George F. Freemesser, M.D., F.A.P.A., C.S.B.

Dr. William Osler wrote, "the human heart has a hidden desire that science cannot satisfy" (1). Many recognize an inner thirst and hunger, emanating from the center of our being, which can only be quenched and satisfied by a broader perception of the world than science can offer.

It is important, however, at the outset to clarify the sense in which we may understand the notion of religion to the satisfaction of all of us. In order to interrelate religion and clinical experience, it is in our best interest to understand religion as nondenominational and within the broadest context, i.e., a belief that there exists a higher power outside ourselves, and, that reality is experienced according to our own individual differences. However, in honesty and fairness, I must admit that whatever I say is influenced by my belief in the Christian faith, as well as a lifetime experience within a specific Christian denomination, the Roman Catholic Church. Furthermore, I wish to acknowledge the profound influence of the Bible on my life.

History reminds us that the relationship between science and religion is characterized by hostility, suspicion, and judgmentalness, but that remains in the past, for hope and wisdom have dawned in a new age. Our journey has taken us a long way from the days when devils had a grip on the world and when Dr. Jonathan Weyer, author of the work *De Praestigius Daemonium*, adamantly rejected all beliefs in witchcraft and strongly condemned all the clergy who supported such beliefs. Dr. Weyer correctly criticized the Church for her penchant to see devils everywhere and for her unsympathetic as well as closed mind to the voice, albeit infant one, of psychiatry, who correctly discerned mental illness as an important factor in the human experience (2).

Great advances have been made in religion and science, and we may now take new steps for mankind in interrelating religion and psychiatry, yet there exists the risk of confusion as we attempt to walk the tightrope of preserving the autonomy of religion and psychology. For those of us who work in the marketplace of therapy, in my view, the most valuable clinical role of religion is to widen our perception of the self, neighbor, and the world. As our age is privileged to see the "*earth rise*," the moon's view of mother earth, so too religion can unfold for clinicians broad new vistas and perceptions, thereby enriching our clinical experience. Such a task is not a luxury, but an urgent need for our survival in the emerging global village world of the 1980s.

Dr. Lawrence Leshan, a humanistic psychologist who is interested in healing, clearly articulates this urgent need when he writes: "One thing is clear, we cannot hope to change our ways of relating to ourselves and others without *major change* in how we *perceive* ourselves and others. It is now imperative that we develop a new and more complete concept of what man is, or we will perish" (3). Clinical experience demonstrates to us, that if our perceptions of the self or neighbor are pessimistic, a positive therapeutic outcome is greatly diminished.

Arnold Toynbee in an overview of history writes, "Man has increased his material power to a degree in which he has become a menace to the biosphere survival. But he has not increased his spiritual potentiality. Man's spiritual potentiality is the only conceivable change in the constitution of the biosphere that can ensure the biosphere and in the biosphere, man himself, against being destroyed by greed that is now armed with the ability to defeat its own intentions" (4).

If we survey the history of the treatment of the mentally ill, there is a note of hope for human beings today to help them face such great changes, vis-à-vis the era of moral treatment, which existed from 1800 to 1850. Great visionaries arose all over the globe to perceive the mentally ill as totally curable, thereby renovating the entire mental health care delivery system. The essence of moral treatment, writes Dr. Ruth Caplan, is "the belief that because of the great malleability of the brain surface, because of its susceptibility to environmental stimuli, pathological conditions could be erased or modified by corrective experience. Insanity, whether a result of direct or indirect injury, or disease, or overwrought emotions, or strained intellectual faculties, could be in every case cured" (5). During the time of my fellowship in general psychiatry at the Mayo Clinic, I was assigned a paper on the evolution of the architectural design of mental hospitals, demonstrating how a change in attitude toward the mentally ill was reflected in the architectural design of the mental hospitals, transforming them from prisonlike structures to homelike buildings. Patients were attended by compassionate and caring people with a fatherly superintendent residing on the hospital grounds, and careful consideration was given to maintaining an optimal ratio between staff and patients. The recovery rates of the moral era have yet to be duplicated in our own age, in spite of the great advancements in technology. Our heads have surged ahead of our hearts in the care of the mentally ill and wounded.

There will be several areas of concerns which we will discuss in this paper and they are as follows:

The Image of the Human Being

The first area of concern regards the image of the human being, that is, the perception of the human being as a total person. As clinicians, we often give lip service to the treatment of the total person; however, in the clinical marketplace, we tend to treat the person as if he or she comes in parts, which is reinforced by an ever-increasing movement toward specialization as well as our tendency to work in isolation. Today, psychosomatic medicine is providing us with new insights of this image; Dr. Z. J. Lypowski writes: "Psychosomatic medicine represents a point of view of the nature of man which affirms that in order to achieve a comprehensive knowledge of people, it is necessary to study man as an individual mind—body complexes, ceaselessly interacting with the social and physical environment in which they are embedded. The psychosomatic concept of man is integrative, holistic and dynamic" (6).

Long before the advent of modern medicine, the Bible, in a holistic manner, always perceived human character in its totality, in words such as these: "one who is cheerful while at table benefits from his food"; "worry has brought death to many"; "envy and anger shorten one's life"; "worry brings on premature old age" (7). Modern medicine teaches us that worry brings on premature aging, such as the effect of the type A personality on heart disease. Furthermore, we have recognized the effect of resentments and grudges as factors in the etiology of cancer, and therefore, if we relate to our patients as bodyless, spiritless minds, then our healing is partial. For example, if we physicians treat heart disease but ignore its psychosocial factors, then only a part of the person is healed. Religion helps us to perceive people as ever changing and maturing, capable of living in two worlds, one that is sense oriented and the other that is spiritually oriented. Secondly, religion provides us with an understanding of human worth and uniqueness, the human role as steward of the created universe as well as individual inner goodness. How urgent and delicate is the task of relating to the total person and not just to behavior. How easily we forget the inner goodness or positiveness of one another as we superficially make judgments based solely on behavior. Religion can assist us in this therapeutic task of coping and balancing the realities of the goodness of the human person and the distortions and pathology of the wounded. The Old Testament powerfully addresses itself to this reality in the words of the prophet Isaiah, "For I am the Lord, your God, the Holy One of Israel, Your Saviour. I give Egypt as your ransom, Ethiopia and Saba in return for you, because you are *precious* in my eyes, glorious, and because *I love you*" (8).

Religion helps us to maintain hope about ourselves in spite of our many failures. The human being is perceived as a wounded individual, who is subject to distortions, difficulties, and failures in personality growth, and in particular, within personal relationships. The prophet Jeremiah writes: "More tortuous than all else is the human heart, beyond remedy, who can understand it? I the Lord alone probe the mind and test the heart" (9). In spite of failures and even stubbornness at times, a remedy is ever available to heal this incurable wound, without denying the painful process but rather utilizing it in moving from woundedness and death toward life and wholeness. Such is the notion of rebirth in religion, that from the womb to the tomb, one grows by a passage from a situation of diminished and/or woundedness toward one of increased life, from one of darkness toward light, from woundedness toward healing; in this manner, then, one continuously matures gradually becoming more whole. The analogy of birth is an excellent model that may help us understand an aspect of our therapeutic work as midwives in assisting people in the move from a more secure (womblike) but diminished life (that is, a defensive, regressive, or distorted one) toward a freer, more autonomous, less defensive lifestyle. Hence, it is through pain and suffering that people grow and increase their lives. Such a perspective may enable us to maintain a more optimistic outlook as well as *patience* in our efforts to assist fellow human beings through the process of rebirth.

But where are we going? What is human maturity? Psychiatry and psychology rarely ask this question and even more rarely study and define the concept of the mature individual. However, there are several people who have addressed themselves to this problem, such as Abraham Maslow, Reza Arasteh, and others. In his book, *Psychology of Being*, Maslow outlines the following characteristics of the mature man: a clear perception of reality, increased wholeness, unity of person, increased spontaneity, firmer identity, creativeness, and ability to adapt.

Reza Arasteh, referring to the notion of the mature individual as "Universal Man," defines human maturity in terms of a person's relationships to others. He includes the following characteristics: kindness to younger people, generosity to the poor, gratitude to teachers, intimacy and trust in friendships; this friendship is best exemplified in the companionship of a congenial, well-suited spouse (10).

Finally, Saint Paul in a powerful, decisive way describes the mature Christian as a new self and a new creation, who is capable of dramatic new behavior, exhibiting mercy, kindness, humility, meekness, patience, ability to bear with other people and forgive others as he/she is forgiven, teaching and admonishing others in terms of psalms, hymns, and spiritual songs, singing one's heart to God (11). Paul categorically states that a drastic change occurs within the inner being of the Christian, which is so profound that the experience seems as if one has died and risen to new life. Having an understanding of human maturity can help us keep our eyes on goals and purposes of the therapeutic process, as well as providing a focus in what can be a confusing process.

The Meaning of Suffering

Pain and suffering are what therapists have to deal with daily, and it is important to consider the various meanings of pain and suffering. In a chapter titled, "The Breakdown of Psychiatry" Dr. Esterson, writes: "Psychiatry makes the assumption that emotional distress is a sign of emotional disorder, that mental breakdown is necessarily harmful and should be stopped as quickly as possible. That madness is primarily the result of something gone wrong inside the person, analogous to a body illness" (12).

As therapists we sometimes find ourselves unable to separate the normal growing pains from the pathological, abnormal ones. There is a tendency to lump everything under the abnormal, which society further reinforces; for example, our society stresses the "happy hour," the serving of depressants to suppress or repress problems rather than encouraging people to deal constructively with them. It appears that our society sees little value in suffering and tries to eliminate its occurrence. There is an ever increasing use of tranquilizers, most of which are prescribed to reduce anxiety, as well as the use of alcohol to suppress the increasing violence in our age. Television is another example of suppressing, often used to pacify various members of society whom we consider problem people, for example, the insane, children, prisoners, mentally sick, aged. In his book *Broken Heart*, Dr. James P. Lynch points out the sad situation of the various intensive care or coronary care units (13). From spending many hours observing doctors and nurses in these acute clinical areas, we have come to recognize that while these individuals spend an extraordinary amount of time with their patients, very little of it is spent simply chatting with them. Almost everything physicians and nurses do is, of necessity, concerned with the patient's illness, rather than with the patient. So even though a great deal of human contact takes place, some patients feel socially isolated and lonely.

While it appears that our age is unable to cope or deal wisely with suffering and pain in the therapeutic process, religion on the other hand is better able to offer us a perspective on suffering that may be more helpful. Pain and suffering can lead to the awareness of the necessity to alter one's lifestyle.

In the book of Exodus, we see such a model with Israel hopelessly enslaved in Egypt, becoming aware of the need for deliverance. God appears to Moses and informs him that He is aware of the affliction of the people of Israel but mysteriously delays their rescue to allow them gradually to become aware of their plight. This delay emphasized a necessary part of the human condition of growth. The same process applies to the alcoholic who must, through long suffering, come to an awareness that he or she has been rendered powerless by alcohol. It is equally true for the neurotic, who must come to that awareness that he or she is entrapped by a neurotic process. Once awareness dawns, it must lead to a decision to change one's lifestyle. The prodigal son in the Bible finally comes to his senses amidst a great deal of turmoil and makes the decision to return home to live a new life. So, too, the alcoholic makes a decision to live a life of sobriety. In the story of Exodus, Israel enters the desert in order to live more freely. In religion the term used for this movement toward a freer life is *metanoia*, which means a conversion or change of one's lifestyle.

Again, awareness is only an initial step, albeit an essential one, in the maturation process. It is the beginning of one's journey toward wholeness or integrity, and for Israel it was the movement into the desert, for the alcoholic into sobriety, and for the neurotic into a less defensive life.

In Paul's Letter to the Hebrews this process of changing one's life is aptly described, and I will summarize: do not grow weary or lose heart, but resist and struggle; be patient and do not lose hope or despair. Paul emphasizes the need for significant others when he writes: "Looking towards the author and finisher of faith, Jesus; to recognize that suffering is part of the discipline of God, meant to correct us and assist us in growth" (14). Similarly in the therapeutic process, the therapist becomes the catalyst. Finally Paul points out that it is only in time that the fruits of the struggle are won, and great patience is required. It is often necessary in the therapeutic process to help one to maintain an attitude of patience and learn not to attempt to accomplish everything all at once. The most vital forces of the therapeutic process are compassion and care, which enable healing to occur, indicating the extent of the therapists' involvement.

There are new forms of compassion, which are now emerging. An article in the *New England Journal of Medicine* refers to the old and new forms of compassion. The old form is an authoritarian one, in which the doctor is the authority and is venerated while the patient is passive and not given any knowledge. In the new form of compassion all are considered partners—doctor, patient, family, and friends. Mutuality is now preferred to one-sidedness (15).

If we are to be more involved in the whole therapeutic process, we must enter into the suffering of the other in order that healing take place. Dr. Lawrence LeShan describes type I healing: "The healer moved into a state of consciousness wherein healer and healee could become totally one, at least for an instant there was no separation in the healer's consciousness. The primary and essential force was love, caring at an intense, deep and profound level. When the process was complete enough, authentic enough, sometimes the healee experienced biological improvement, the healer often felt better, not drained or weakened in any sense" (16).

Healing requires intimate involvement with the wounded rather than an objective distance. However, in order to cure, one cannot remain at a distance; to be a healer is to be intimately involved in a caring manner. It is caring through *being with* rather than *doing to* another. The experience of *being with* someone is foreign to the Western activist's mental attitude. However, we now understand that techniques, no matter how many and varied, or our own theoretical approaches are of lesser importance than the care and trust in our therapeutic relationships. So often our therapeutic attempts are frustrated because the personal qualities of the therapist take a backseat in the therapeutic armatorium. Far too often control exceeds care.

Underground Madness

In the modern, technological age such as ours, the pace tends to be hectic, energy expenditure enormous, anxiety pervasive. People exhibit obsessive preoccupation with success and achievement, and a consistent over-stimulation of the aggressive drive is a direct consequence of multitudinous pressures. The type A personality (17), now known to be associated with heart disease and premature death, leads to intense over-stimulation of the sympathetic nervous system, resulting in expending energy as well as increased aggressive feelings, which are in our culture repressed rather than expressed. This repression means that resentments and angers accumulate within the individual, dramatically influencing a modern person's lifestyle, which is characterized by an acceleration of common activity, a feeling of time urgency, a struggle against the limitation of time, a tenseness of facial musculature, a restlessness, and an explosiveness of speech, all included within the type A personality. A common signpost of repression is tension, which often leads to escape in excessive activity; furthermore, the most significant effect of type A personality is that of interpersonal isolation and alienation. Dr. Rollo May writes about the cultural meaning of anxiety in his book *Individual Competitive Success Syndrome*, and he demonstrates how a person can become rapidly entangled in a vicious circle of anxiety, described in the following manner:

COMPETITIVE STRIVING

INCREASED ANXIETY   *INTRASOCIAL HOSTILITY*

INTERPERSONAL ISOLATION

Furthermore, competitive success is not essentially a matter of achieving material security, nor is it in the realm of sex and love, a matter of achieving an abundance of libidinal satisfaction. Rather, continues May, it is a matter of gaining security because it is accepted as a proof of one's power in one's own eyes and in the eyes of others (18). In a sense, economic evaluation becomes valuations of persons, hence we relate to one another as *competitors*, rather than as *cooperators*. This relationship finally creates an atmosphere of suspicion between one another, resulting in intense feelings of interpersonal isolation and alienation. Insofar as we repress resentments, self-pity, guilt, mistrust, etc., there exist barriers between ourselves and the person against whom we hold these inner negative feelings. It is underground madness or grudge-sludge; that is, the person is mad at self, at neighbor, and at the world. The recent developments in psychosomatic medicine now view and understand repressed emotions as serious factors in all medical illnesses; however, there is little known about how to treat and heal the illnesses resulting from such repressed emotions.

As a psychiatrist, I have felt discouraged and helpless for many years in regard to the healing of repressed emotions, particularly that of repressed resentments; it is so much easier to assist someone in coping with anger or aggression within interpersonal relationships, but once the resentment is repressed, healing is extremely difficult. People have a powerful tendency to hold on to revenges and grudges for even many years' duration. In my view, only religion offers hope to assist us in healing such repressed emotions because only religion can help us understand the reality of forgiveness in its totality, which includes not only forgiveness, but also *forgetting* or healing. It is a common human experience to be able to forgive one another rather easily, but one is not able to forget the hurts and resentments; we hold on to the memory of our hurts, using it as a weapon against our neighbor. When we try to forget these bad memories, we feel helpless and hopeless, and then religion offers us a new hopeful perspective of healing. It requires healing of every hurt, resentment, or negative memory in order for two people to be fully reconciled. Without the healing, the forgetting of all hurtful memories, there can be no reestablishment of communication between two people, that is, a total reconciliation.

An analogy that may enlighten us regarding such phenomena as retained memories is that of an abscess. In the physical sense an abscess manifests itself in generalized symptoms that include chills, fever, and fatigue. So, too, with the psychological or spiritual abscess, which manifests itself by increased irritability, especially in the presence of the irritant or the person against whom the feelings are held. The result is an underlying solidification or bitterness, isolation, and loneliness. Hence there is a need to drain such an inner abscess in order to allow the healing process to take place. Alcoholics Anonymous has long recognized such phenomena and takes steps to eradicate these realities, especially in several of the well-known twelve steps in the Alcoholics Anonymous program. On several of these steps, there is referral to recognizable injuries, wounds, and memories of hurts that have been done to other people throughout the long, destructive process of alcoholism, as well as the need for forgiveness to take place. Several of the steps require that a list of faults and hurts against other people be drawn up, as well as a list of people to be forgiven; the alcoholic deals with such a list with the help of another trusted person.

In recent years, as a priest, I have experienced powerful healings and have witnessed many healings take place during the relieving of such grudges, hurts, and bitternesses through the utilization of imaginative techniques, very similar to those used by Dr. Carl Simonton in Fort Worth, Texas, in the psychotherapy of cancer. The healing technique is called the "Healing of Memories," in which a survey of one's whole life is made in order to become aware of the presence of hurtful memories that have accumulated throughout the years and are still exerting their effect on the personality. Then, through the use of imagination one meets Jesus of Nazareth, who shares the fullness of his forgiveness as God to eradicate and heal all these memories and requires the individual to share that same forgiveness with all those who have hurt him or her. Furthermore, I have discovered that intercessory prayer and fasting are excellent techniques for the purification, not only of the body but also for the eradication of many negative memories, grudge-sludge, or underground madness. I often ask my patients to fast for the person against whom they hold these grudges or by whom they have been wounded and find in almost every case a healing of the inner resentments as well as a stimulation of more positive caring and warm feelings for that person who was originally an enemy. Through the use of intercessory prayer, focus is given toward the wounded individual, and it is impossible to hold negative affect against someone for whom you are praying. Hence, the negative feelings are healed and positive feelings are stimulated toward the resented person. Furthermore, I also use this technique with my own patients, especially when we come to a therapeutic standstill or impasse; through mutual fasting we often experience a great breakthrough. In my experience the healing of memories often is felt on a physiological level with definite decrease in muscular tension, a lowering of blood pressure, slowing of heart rate, and the like.

Community—Toward a Healing Community

The last area to be considered is the most important one—that of community. It is my contention that as caregivers if we do not learn to work together as a community, we cannot survive in the future. All of us should ask ourselves questions: Who takes care of me, the caregiver? Who nurtures the nurturer? Usually the answer is silence followed by more silence.

The essential aspect of community, on my group or teamwork, is the element of ministering to one another. It seems to me that in the future we can no longer work in isolation as we do currently, nor can we continue to work without ministering or nurturing one another, for the burdens of caregiving become heavier and heavier as technology rapidly advances. As long as we follow competitive molds, we shall devour one another and be devoured, thereby diminishing our healing power and depleting our caring energies. As was pointed out earlier in reference to new modes of compassion, we understand that the competitive, authoritative model of medical practice, so frequently utilized in modern health care systems, is now outdated and outmoded. Within the newer form of compassion, ever so gradually emerging, friends, family, and the caregivers become mutual partners rather than relating to one another in a unilateral, hierarchical, authoritative manner. The key words to describe this phenomena are sharing, caring, and cooperating, rather than possessing, competing, and remaining aloof. Hence, religion may open a whole new perspective in regards to the notion of community, for it forces us to view ourselves as members of one family. Religion reinforces the notion that we are indeed our brother's keeper, and it is a part of our duty as fellow human beings to share, care, and bear the burdens of each other. May underscores a new sense of community when he writes about compassion in these words: "Compassion is that form of love which is based on our knowing and our understanding each other. Compassion is the awareness that we are all in the same boat, that we all shall either sink or swim together. Compassion arises from the recognition of community. It realizes that all men and women are brothers and sisters, even though a disciplining of our instincts is necessary for us to even begin to carry out that belief in our actions" (19).

In the opinion of this author, our world is at a crucial point in its history so that this lesson, if not learned, will lead to very destructive and disruptive effects in our whole global village as well as in the caregiving field. I feel so strongly about the development of this new sense of community within the health-care system, that I am willing to make such bold statements.

Furthermore, the human body offers us a superb analogy as well as wisdom about the possible organization of a community of human persons based on a similar organization of a community of cells within the human body. It is known that the health of the whole body depends on the health of each of the individual cells and that this health is true is so dramatically demonstrated in the fact that cancer, which may destroy the whole body, is initiated by just one cell. Similarly, in a community of persons, the health of the body of common humanity depends upon the willingness of each of the individual members to share their vitality, i.e., their resources, with one another. Furthermore, so intimate is the union among all of us, that if we do not share our vitalities, we do a disservice to all humanity as well as to our individual selves. This statement is a strong one about the importance of community life, and it is a powerful declaration about individual worth. How important it is to develop an understanding that each of us as an individual can infect the entire global village, yet this thought is contrary to the very strong sense of individualism prevalent in our North American culture.

In summary, then, we try to look at religion not from a denominational viewpoint but rather from the viewpoint of new perspectives enabling us to enlarge and increase our options in the care-giving field. First of all, we try to see how religion may enlarge our understanding of the image of the human being so that it will lead us to a much more optimistic therapeutic approach toward the total person and people with whom we work. Secondly, we consider the phenomena of forgiveness and repression of emotions and how religion might assist us in understanding a new perspective of forgetting and healing such repressed emotions. Lastly, we consider the notion of community and what effect this notion might have upon the future of the care-giving field.

May our hearts then be open to new vistas enabling us to see new visions, dream new dreams, and hope for new possibilities in the vital work of care giving. As we have witnessed the earth rise, the moon's view of mother earth, may we now experience an uplifting of our spirits, a fresh new vision that allows us to care for our fellows in a healing manner.

References

1. Sederer, Lloyd. "Moral Therapy and Problem of Morale," *American Journal of Psychiatry* 134: 3, March 1977, p. 267.

2. Weyer, Johann. *De Praestigius Daemonium, Comprehensive Textbook of Psychiatry, II*. Alfred M. Freedman, Harold Kaplan, & Benjamin Sadock (eds.). Baltimore: Williams & Wilkins Co., 1975, p. 34.

3. Goodrick, Joyce. "Healing Implications for Psychotherapy." In Fosshage (ed.). New York: Humanistic Science Press, 1978, p. 86.

4. Toynbee, Arnold. *Mother Earth and Mankind*. New York and London: Oxford University Press, 1976, p. 575.

5. Caplan, Ruth. *Psychiatry and the Community in Nineteenth Century America*. New York: Basic Books, 1969, p. 26.

6. Lipowski, Z. J. "Psychosomatic Medicine in the Seventies: An Overview." *American Journal of Psychiatry* 134: 3, March 1977, p. 234.

7. Holy Bible, St. Joseph New Catholic Edition, Douay Version. New York: Catholic Publishing Co., 1962. Sirach Chapter 30.

8. Ibid., Isaiah 43: 103–104.

9. Ibid., Jeremiah 17: 9.

10. Arasteh, Reza. *Final Integration of the Adult Personality*. Leiden, Netherlands: E. J. Briu, 1965, pp. 139–140.

11. Holy Bible, Collosians 3: 12, 14, 16.

12. Esterson, M. D. "Healing, Implications for Psychotherapy." Chapter 13, p. 352.

13. Lynch, James. *Broken Heart*. New York: Basic Books, 1977, p. 151.

14. Holy Bible, Hebrews 12: 1–15.

15. Barber, Bernard. "Seminars in Medicine of the Beth Israel Hospital." *New England Journal of Medicine*, 298 (77), October 1976, p. 931.

16. Esterson, "Healing Implications for Psychotherapy," p. 90.

17. Jenkins, C. David, Rosenman, Ray H., & Zysanski, Stephen J. "Prediction of Clinical Coronary Heart Disease by a test for the Coronary-prone Behavior Pattern." *The New England Journal of Medicine* 290, (23), June 6, 1974, p. 1271.

18. May, Rollo. *The Meaning of Anxiety*. New York: Ronald Press Company, 1950, pp. 181–183.

19. May, Rollo. *Power and Innocence*. New York: W. W. Norton Co., 1972, p. 251.

TIPs: A Preventive Mental Health Model for Parenting Education

Mary Wanda Draper, Ph.D.

TIPs (toddlers, infants, and parents) was developed as a model for preventive parenting education and child development. The program, designed to promote preventive mental health services and education, was implemented in 1976, under the leadership of the author. The TIPs model was conceived as a practical effort to meet the ongoing challenge of putting into action the philosophically and rhetorically based priority so often placed on prevention.

The Challenge of Prevention

Preventive mental health may well be the least understood and the most neglected area of public health in our nation. Basic to the notion of preventive mental health is the belief that we can have an improved future quality of life by giving attention to individuals and families before serious problems and disturbances occur. Science has demonstrated this concept with a record of more progress in prevention supportive of physical health than any other sphere related to human development.

Prevention has two distinct focuses. The first is a thrust for protection against those impacting forces that contribute to poor mental health such as societal and environmental obstacles, lack of personal knowledge and skills, and vulnerability to the stresses of daily living. Preventive action is aimed at avoiding the onset of poor mental health by anticipating and dealing with the causes of problems before they afflict the individual or family. Crisis prevention and anticipatory guidance are based upon the premise that a significant amount of pain, misery, agony, and unhappiness can be averted by actions designed to improve coping skills while reducing levels of frustration, anxiety, and stress.

A second thrust involves a systematic delivery of services that assures the promotion and continuity of positive mental health. This effort includes such avenues as providing for the needs of children in the context of their families and communities and requires structuring services around the child and family instead of attempting to provide them through numerous agencies.

Prevention is aimed at keeping families intact. Needed is a unified system of services that makes it as easy for families to go to a community center for assistance in preventing problems as to an emergency room after problems have become serious and disruptive to individual or family life. Ideally, prevention aims at eliminating the need to go to either of these.

Kenneth Keniston and The Carnegie Council on Children, in their 1977 edition of *All Our Children*, describes the American parent as being caught up in the midst of change in today's world and reflects the need for preventive services and education.

> American parents today are worried and uncertain about how to bring up their children. They feel unclear about the proper balance between permissiveness and firmness. They fear they are neglecting their children, yet sometimes resent the demands their children make. Americans wonder whether they are doing a good job as parents, yet are unable to define just what a good job is. In droves, they seek expert advice. And many prospective parents wonder whether they ought to have children at all.
>
> None of this is altogether new or uniquely American. —What is new and very American is the intensity of the malaise, the sense of having no guidelines or supports for raising children, the feeling of not being in control as parents, and the widespread sense of personal guilt for what seems to be going awry. For when the right way to be a parent is not clear, almost any action can seem capricious or wrong, and every little trouble or minor storm in one's children's lives can become the cause for added self-blame.

A false assumption seems to prevail in America that parents are solely responsible for the upbringing of their children and for the success of family life. Parents and their children are constantly bombarded by societal pressures from outside the family unit. They need support systems that provide encouragement and assistance in handling conflict and dealing with uncertainties of everyday life. Parents need help in identifying and considering alternatives as they meet the challenges that await them.

The issue of prevention deals less with the cost of rendering adequate mental health care to all children than with how much will be saved by serving needy children and families who are headed for trouble. Promoting mental health for children before they become adults not only decreases the probability of later problems but also saves in the cost of treatment and rehabilitation. Two examples cited by Zigler and Hunsinger (1979) demonstrate the need to reorder priorities in terms of action aimed at prevention.

> While the federal government spends nearly $250 million a year to maintain children in foster care, very little money is directed toward services that might prevent family breakup or promote family reunification. Yet, demonstration projects show that given adequate homemaker and other social services during times of crisis, a large percentage of family breakups and related foster care placements can be avoided.
> While the federal government has sponsored some innovative community services to combat child abuse, these programs are few in number and limited to after-the-fact services rather than prevention of abuse before it occurs.

The underlying premise of the TIPs program is that beginning with children will ultimately have benefits for all ages. A preventive approach that serves children more appropriately will, by its very nature, be more efficacious in serving adults.

The TIPs Model

Purpose

The overall purpose of TIPs is fourfold: (1) to establish a model delivery system for preventive mental health in the areas of parenting and child development, (2) to provide preventive education for child rearing, (3) to enhance children's overall development through stimulation and enrichment experiences for infants and toddlers, and (4) to provide education in preventive mental health to professional trainees.

The focus for the parents is on increasing competencies for parenting through affirming healthy attitudes about themselves as individuals and as parents, expanding their knowledge of child development, and developing skills in child rearing. For the infants and toddlers the focus is on providing a wholesome and supportive atmosphere for sensory and motor stimulation and social interaction through spontaneous play experiences.

Parents participating in the TIPs programs expressed initial concerns that fall into three general categories: (1) a desire to learn more about what is normal development for their children, (2) what to expect as children progress from one stage of development to the next, and (3) how to exercise effective guidance and discipline.

Philosophy

The TIPs philosophy supports the premise that parents are the most significant influence on their children's lives and therefore are their most effective teachers. Although the professionals interact with the children during the TIPs activities, the overall approach of the program is that the professional works with the parent and the parent works with the child.

Emphasis is placed on acceptance and affirmation of oneself as a parent who has a broad range of personal needs and interests that include, but go beyond, parenting. Underlying the activities are three concerns: (1) developing meaningful relationships between parent and child, (2) enjoyment of infants and toddlers, and (3) the importance of nurturance and support, especially during the first three years of the child's life.

Staff

The child development specialist, on the child psychiatry outpatient clinic faculty, serves as the TIPs consultant, providing leadership for the overall program. Professional trainees in the child psychiatry program provide child development assistance by working with the infants and toddlers. These trainees consist of medical students, child psychiatry fellows, general psychiatry residents, psychology and psychiatric social work interns, and special education practicum students. The trainees are scheduled on a rotation basis so that two to three persons work with the children during each TIPs meeting. Child psychiatrists, psychologists, social workers, and education specialists on the faculty lend support to the program as needed.

Four family advocates, employed as staff personnel in the Child and Family Resource Program also serve as child development assistants. One or two advocates are present for each session. The advocates and professional trainees work together to serve as models for interacting with the infants and toddlers and for facilitating stimulation and enrichment activities.

Format for Program Activities

Parents, bringing their infants and toddlers with them, began to participate in the TIPs program at the child psychiatry outpatient clinic in the fall of 1976. The program began as a joint effort between the Department of Psychiatry and Behavioral Sciences and the Child and Family Resource Program (CFRP), one of eleven federally funded demonstration projects in the nation. CFRP participants represent rural and suburban low-income families in the eastern vicinity of the greater Oklahoma City area. The ages of parents range from 17 to 30 years, while children's ages range from newborns to 36 months.

Parents and their children attend the TIPs activities during the morning every other week for six months. Each meeting consists of three hours of activities. While the schedule is flexible to meet family needs, the following format serves as a basis for the program.

Parent-child interaction time. During the first segment of the morning, parents and their children interact together in a large playroom while TIPs staff observe them through an adjoining observation booth for about a half hour. This activity gives parents an opportunity to help their children settle in and become familiar with the playroom and child development assistants who remain with the children throughout the morning. The viewing time provides an opportunity for the TIPs staff and professional trainees to observe parent behaviors and child-rearing practices as well as developmental stages characteristic of each child. These observations provide implications for subsequent discussions with parents concerning principles of development, parent attitudes, and interaction styles. Feedback to the child development assistants also strengthens their efforts as role models for subsequent sessions. This beginning activity also sets parents at ease for getting acquainted with each other and the assistants in an informal way while sharing ideas and concerns about their children.

Parent and staff observation period. Following the first half hour with their children, parents move from the playroom to the observation booth where they experience a view of their children from a distance, through a one-way vision window. The TIPs consultant serves as the mediator during this period, describing and pointing out subtle as well as explicit indicators of development. This informal period allows parents to ask questions about their children's behavior and development and to make comments.

The booth interaction serves multiple purposes. Parents often express feelings and anxieties about their children's actions or about their tasks as parents. They ask questions about what their children are doing at the moment. Parents get immediate feedback about their concerns. They are also stimulated to share ideas and to express their feelings about what they see. Parental responses and questions, while viewing their children, provide valuable implications for planning TIPs discussions and ongoing activities. They also learn by watching the modeling behavior of the staff with the children in the playroom. Modeling objectives include demonstrating caring and nurturing attitudes and responses to the children, practicing nonpunitive techniques of setting limits and guiding behavior, and enhancing development by facilitating children's active involvement with other persons, toys, and materials.

Parent discussion group meetings. Following the observation period the TIPs consultant and parents meet in a group to talk about child development and parenting concerns. Discussions center around such topics as parent-child relationships, health care and safety, nutrition, intellectual and language development, social skills, emotional development, clothing that promotes or hinders development, learning through play. Although a given topic is planned for each meeting, parents' immediate concerns are given priority. For example, when a parent has a problem concerning a child such as excessive biting behavior, this is discussed before taking up the planned topic of the day. This approach further supports the TIPs philosophy that immediate feedback relative to personal experiences and issues enhances learning while keeping the focus on the parents and their children rather than on the curriculum or the program itself.

The group size of ten to twelve parents lends to active participation of each person in the discussion group. The consultant's objective is to provide a climate for creative learning through group interplay in which each parent feels free to express ideas and concerns without fear of rejection or ridicule. Although the consultant provides leadership for dealing with content information and feedback, the group is encouraged to share actively in the learning process. In this context, the ultimate objective for the parents is the unleashing of their potentialities and strengths that make it possible for them to broaden their own spectrum of options for handling conflict and dealing with problems and incongruencies.

Following the discussion period the parents return to the playroom for a few minutes of interaction with their children prior to departure. During the discussion period parents may see about their children should they feel the need.

Developmental kits. Each time the parents meet they are provided with a kit of toys to take home for use during the two-week interim. The TIPs consultant discusses the toys and their value for children at various stages of development. The primary objective of the kits is to stimulate parent and child interaction in the home setting. Upon returning to the TIPs meetings, parents bring their kits in exchange for the next kits to be used.

Hot line. During the first project year an automatic answering service was installed in the child development specialist's office to allow parents to call in day or night to register particular problems or concerns related to child rearing. The calls were answered by faculty or trainees during the subsequent twenty-four hour period. The idea in using the hot line was to prevent potential problems before they became serious and to help parents try alternatives to child-rearing tasks.

Home visits. Upon request, or out of obvious need, the CFRP advocates visit the homes of TIPs families to maintain rapport and provide encouragement and assistance. The assistance may be related to child development and parenting or it may vary to include such help as providing information about job opportunities, welfare assistance, and consumer assistance. This service further supports a preventive approach.

Evaluation

The evaluation component for the TIPs model consists of (1) a general assessment of overall program effectiveness, (2) interviews with participating parents, and (3) a research component designed to measure change in attitudes and knowledge of parents in relation to child rearing.

General assessment

A debriefing session for the professional trainees and the family advocates at the conclusion of each TIPs meeting provides feedback regarding the morning's activities and input for improving future meetings. Parental attitudes toward and participation in the educational process are considered as well as such aspects as effectiveness of the trainees with the infants and toddlers, implications from observations, the use of developmental kits, and the group interplay during discussion periods. These data are used in making adjustments in emphasis on topics for discussion, in efforts to improve modeling behaviors with the children, and in making other changes to improve the effectiveness of the experiences for both parents and children.

Interviews with Parents

Each parent agreed to participate in an interview at the conclusion of the TIPs program series. The interview consists of an inventory of 45 questions developed by the child development consultant, two child psychiatry fellows, and the family advocates. The interview questions are aimed at getting a closer look at (1) how each participant conceptualizes himself or herself as a parent, (2) their behavior patterns in relating to children, and (3) knowledge and attitudes about parenting.

The family advocates received training from the child development specialist and child psychiatry fellows in conducting the interviews. Using the questions on the inventory, the advocates role-played the positions of parent and interviewer in an effort to develop sensitivity to parents and to be able to frame the questions in a meaningful way. This process was videotaped for self study and to improve the questions and techniques prior to administering the questionnaire to the parents. Each parent was interviewed by one of the family advocates. The interviews were recorded and videotaped for transcription of exact responses and for use in studying body language, voice tonality, and general responsiveness of parents.

Implications for further program development were derived from the data as well as greater insights into the actual parental behaviors reflected by parent responses.

Research Design

A research component was designed during the first year of TIPs, therefore data were not collected and measured for the subjects in the pilot program. Data gathering and analysis began with the subsequent year's program.

Hypotheses. Two major hypotheses were formulated: that the TIPs experience would effect a significant change in attitudes toward child guidance on the part of the participating parents and that the TIPs experience would significantly increase the child development knowledge base of participating parents.

Subjects. Subjects for the TIPs research formed two groups: *experimental*, those parents participating in the TIPs program, and *control*, those parents (selected on a matching basis with the experimental subjects) who did not participate in the program.

Instrumentation. Two instruments were used to collect data: The Inventory of Attitudes on Child Guidance, by McKinzie (revised) and The Parent Knowledge Inventory, by Draper and Draper (revised).

Pre- and post-tests were administered to the experimental and control group subjects prior to the TIPs program and after its completion.

Statistical treatment. A two-way analysis of variance was selected as the statistic to treat the data for ascertaining changes in parental attitudes and knowledge, respectively. The .05 level of significance was selected as a basis for supporting or rejecting the hypotheses inasmuch as this was an exploratory study.

Changes Made to Improve the Model

Second Year

Three major changes were implemented during the second year of TIPs. First, the location of the program was changed from the child psychiatry outpatient clinic to the local CFRP center. The parents brought their children to the CFRP center in their own community instead of traveling to Oklahoma City. The CFRP facility was renovated to include an infant-toddler playroom with an adjoining observation room that also served as the center for parent discussion sessions. This change in location was more realistic for supporting the program as an integral part of community activities. The CFRP and the local Head Start program share the same physical facility. This change accommodated parents and their families, especially those with preschool and elementary-age children.

The second change was to shift the major responsibility for facilitating and coordinating the program to the CFRP family advocates, with the child development specialist now serving as a consultant to provide training and technical assistance to the advocates. To serve as a training model, the consultant continued to play a major role in leading the discussion groups during the second year. These changes were a successful attempt to make the TIPs program more of an integral part of the broader CFRP.

The third change was to discontinue the automatic telephone answering service. This change reduced the cost of operating the program and placed more responsibility on the advocates for responding to the needs of parents. The advocates' telephone numbers were available to the parents. Many parents reported that they discussed their problems and concerns in the TIPs discussion group meetings, in home visits, or with each other.

Third Year

In its third year the TIPs program continued with one additional activity designed to upgrade the competencies and skills of the family advocates in providing more effective leadership for the program. A series of six child development seminars was conducted by the child development consultant. The advocates assumed the responsibility for planning and leading the discussion groups as well as for coordinating the entire program. This change strengthened the TIPs program as part of the CFRP community and enhanced the self-images of the family advocates. The child development specialist only serves as a consultant to the program.

Exporting the Model

In the summer of 1978, the child development consultant directed a TIPs training program for sixteen secondary public school teachers from various parts of Oklahoma. The purpose of the training was to prepare teachers of child development and family life education to implement TIPs programs in their respective communities as part of their vocational adult education programs in the public schools. Faculty in the child psychiatry outpatient clinic, including child psychiatrists, psychologists, child development specialists, and social workers provided workshops to assist the teachers in upgrading their teaching skills in parenting and child development and to develop a plan to involve parents and their children in TIPs programs.

At the time of this writing, twelve teachers have implemented programs in both rural and urban areas reaching over 120 parents and over 150 children that represent a cross section of socioeconomic and ethnic strata in all quadrants of the state.

The TIPs model was implemented with minor variations to accommodate the particular and unique situations in the respective communities. For example, programs that have no observation facilities use a "modeling and discussion" approach while in the playroom. The teacher talks with the parents informally while they interact with their children. High school students participate as child care assistants while the parents meet with the teacher for their discussion group activities.

These teachers, during their 1979 annual vocational education conference, met with the child development consultant for a brief evaluation of progress and to discuss the research component. The teachers reported enthusiasm on the part of the parents and the assisting high school students. Several teachers plan to continue the TIPs programs as an ongoing part of their adult education curriculum. Many of the participants are school-age parents who have one or two infants.

Data are being gathered on a pre- and post-test basis for all the vocational TIPs subjects and for matching control subjects. Using the above research design, two child psychiatry fellows under the supervision of the child development specialist are in the process of analyzing the data for the statewide TIPs effort.

Conclusions

The TIPs program appears to reflect favorable progress toward meeting its purposes as a model for preventive mental health in areas of parenting and child development. Parent responses related to what they derived from the program also reflect progress toward achieving program objectives. The responses most reported, in order of frequency include:

Fewer feelings of guilt as a parent who cannot do everything.

Having more fun with children.

Knowing what to expect that is normal in the child's development.

More patience; less spanking; less yelling at children.

Less frustration when things go wrong.

Less dependency on others for help.

Several advantages benefit the TIPs program. The same child development specialist continued to work with the program from the outset; a multidisciplinary faculty support system strengthened the basis of the program; professional trainees provided valuable input while receiving practical training; application of the research component placed the hypothetical assumptions under the scrutiny of statistical treatment and analysis; and collaboration with community-based programs required a realistic perspective that called for implementing changes to meet current situational needs.

The TIPs program portrays an evolving and realistic approach to working with parents and their young children in supportive and nonthreatening ways. The programs center around meeting the particular needs and interests of each participating parent and child. TIPs promotes the notion that a society that supports its children, its most valuable and also most vulnerable resource, is a society that strengthens its future. We have a choice of being *history menders* or *history benders*; TIPs aims at accomplishing the latter.

References

Brazelton, T. Berry. *Infants and Mothers*. New York: Delacorte Press/ Seymour Lawrence, 1969.

Brazelton, T. Berry. *Toddlers and Parents*. New York: Delacorte Press/Seymour Lawrence, 1974.

Draper, H. E., & Draper, M. W. "Study of the Cognitive and Affective Domains of Students Studying Child Development." University of Wisconsin-Stout, 1970.

Draper, M. W., & Draper, H. E. *Caring for Children*. Peoria: Charles A. Bennett Co., 1979.

Keniston, Kenneth, & The Carnegie Council on Children. *All Our Children*. New York: Harcourt Brace Jovanovich, 1977.

U.S. Department of Health, Education, and Welfare Public Health Service. *Primary Prevention: An Idea Whose Time Has Come*. National Institute of Mental Health, 1977.

White, Burton. *The First Three Years of Life*. Englewood Cliffs, N.J.: Prentice-Hall, 1975.

Zigler, Edward, & Hunsinger, Susan. "Look at the State of America's Children in the Year of the Child." *Young Children*, January 1979.

Social and Cultural Factors in the Delivery of Mental Health Services

Wayne H. Holtzman, Ph.D.

Notable changes in the amount and variety of services for people with mental and emotional problems have occurred during the past thirty years. Some differences have come in the type of care given and in the location of such services. The establishment of the National Institute of Mental Health in 1948 marked the beginning of a new era. Robert H. Felix, the first director of NIMH, started with a budget of only $4 million and several offices from the U.S. Public Health Service.

Twenty-five years and $4.3 billion later, one of his successors, Bertram S. Brown (1973), pointed to a number of remarkable changes in state mental hospitals, community mental health centers, the kinds of mental health services offered, and the great increase in numbers of mental health professionals who offer services. The number of residents in state mental hospitals dropped from a high of a half-million in 1955 to only 275,000 in 1972. The expenditure per patient day increased from only $1.81 in 1948 to $20.68 over this same period.

Thirty years ago there were five resident-patients for each full-time staff member in contrast to the current ratio in which the number of staff members is almost equal to the number of patients. More important has been the sharp drop in length of hospitalization from an average of more than six months to a median length of stay of just forty-one days for 1972 admissions.

A dramatic shift in the locus and type of care during the past quarter-century has also occurred. In 1955 one-half of the nearly two million episodes of care were provided by the traditional public mental hospitals. Twenty years later only 9 percent of the 6.4 million episodes were accounted for by state and county mental hospitals. Nearly one-half of today's therapy is provided by outpatient psychiatric services, while almost another one-third takes place in community mental health centers. As the President's Commission on Mental Health pointed out (1978), the greatest changes have been the increase of the elderly in nursing homes, the marked shift from mental institutions to community care facilities, and the rise in treatment of alcohol-related disorders in mental institutions. Many factors are responsible for these changes, and several stand out as particularly noteworthy.

Gerald L. Klerman, former head of the Alcohol, Drug Abuse, and Mental Health Administration, has described two professional developments that occurred almost simultaneously in the mid-1950s revolutionizing the treatment of schizophrenia and other mental illnesses (1977). The first of the so-called tranquilizers, rauwolfia and the phenothiazines, contributed to improved treatment of many acute psychotic patients. The second major development involved new psychosocial and behavioral methods of treatment in the mental hospital, leading to new social reform. These quite different developments—the biomedical and the psychosocial—continue to stimulate debate and controversy concerning the ultimate answers to the still-baffling problems of diagnosis and treatment of the mentally ill. Whether one is conducting work on the new frontiers of neurohormones and behavior in a search for better medical treatment or whether one is engaged in new experiments with social organization and the technologies of behavior modification, the delivery of mental health services must be pressed forward vigorously without waiting for future developments.

Several models of care demonstrate changing philosophies. In the first pattern, emphasis is upon the professional expert's engaging in diagnosis and treatment of a mental illness. This is the medical model. Here the clinical skills of the professional and his assistants are of paramount importance in providing effective services for the person in need of help. Close attention must be paid to environmental-behavioral interactions within the family as well as in the cultural milieu in order to be effective, in most cases.

A second approach grows out of the preventative model championed by public health. Here the strategy is one of locating the focal points in society where high risk of emotional breakdown can be determined and then developing social practices that are aimed at minimizing the degree of mental illness that occurs. A primary focus is upon illness and its prevention.

The third point of view has sometimes been called the positive mental health approach. Its emphasis is on large-scale educational and social intervention in order to overcome cultural and environmental factors that prevent the full development of an individual's potential.

The community movement places strong emphasis upon a combination of preventative health measures and social intervention aimed at promoting greater mental health. Clinical services tend to be short-term for crisis intervention. The professional devotes more of his time to preparing others (such as parents and teachers) to deal with the problems themselves rather than offering to deal directly with the problems of others. All the models represent valid approaches. Each pattern also has serious limitations that are overlooked all too often.

The Community Mental Health Movement

A broad consensus was reached across the land following the reports of the Joint Commission on Mental Illness and Health in 1961. The Commission's final report placed strong emphasis on community-based services, leading to the Mental Retardation Facilities and Community Mental Health Centers Construction Act of 1963. The Association of Psychiatric Outpatient Centers of America was formed at this same time. Swept up in the ambitious federal program of Kennedy's New Frontier and Johnson's Great Society, the community mental health movement was born in a climate of enthusiasm and hope for the future.

In 1977 some 726 community mental health centers throughout the country received federal funding totaling more than a quarter-billion dollars per year. The $1.5 billion in categorical federal funding during the first fifteen years of the community mental health center program attracted nearly $5 billion of additional support from non-federal sources. Useful mental health projects have been introduced in hundreds of communities where there would be few or no services if the federal program had not produced them. In spite of these great gains, serious problems remain throughout the country with regard to delivering mental health services. As the President's Commission on Mental Health (1978) noted, many areas still have virtually no mental health programs while others suffer from major deficiencies for large segments of the population. Even where well-established centers exist, a distressing lack of service is too often evident for the after-care of mental patients who are returning to the community.

Additional federal legislation passed by Congress in 1975 revised substantially the original Community Mental Health Centers Act. The 1975 legislation defined for the first time what comprehensive mental health services must be provided by a community mental health center in order to qualify for federal assistance. With passage of new legislation under the Reagan administration in 1981 federal assistance shifted from categorical funding through NIMH to funding through block grants to the states at a reduced level. The five core services essential to a comprehensive center are emergency care, both outpatient and inpatient care, partial hospitalization, and some form of consultation and educational activity for others in the community. Seven additional services are also recommended to deal with children, the elderly, court-screening, follow-up care for ex-patients, transitional living facilities, and the treatment of alcoholism and drug abuse.

In only a few community mental health centers are all of these services effectively rendered in a comprehensive manner for the entire community. All too frequently the limited funds and lack of direction preclude the continuum of services from crisis intervention to after-care support originally envisioned fifteen years ago. As the President's Commission stated, many people with chronic mental illness have no choice but to live in cheap rooming houses or nursing homes ill equipped to serve them. Many persons would be better off remaining under institutional care where, at least, humane treatment would be offered.

A point noted by the 1975 federal legislation and repeatedly stressed by the Commission is the extent to which large segments of our population continue to be underserved. Populations especially at risk were recognized in this most recent legislation—children and youth, the elderly, and substance abusers. It was also apparent to anyone who closely examined the uneven distribution of services that programs aimed at helping minorities and the poor had fallen far short of their initial goals.

When services are available, all too frequently they conflict with the cultural or linguistic traditions of ethnic minorities and the urban poor. It is worth noting that fewer than 2 percent of all psychiatrists in America are black, while the percentage of Spanish-speaking psychiatrists is even lower. Among the traditional professions, only social work and nursing show any appreciable increase in minorities over the past ten years.

For these reasons, the newly proposed Mental Health Systems Act was given high priority by President Carter's administration. This new program would have shifted emphasis from large comprehensive service centers to discrete services most urgently needed to serve especially vulnerable populations, if it had not been rendered moot by subsequent legislation. This new look within community mental health would require close attention to social and cultural factors underlying delivery of mental health services in the country. Among the many such factors are several that tend to be underplayed in spite of their importance. The first of these is the family.

Family Environment and Mental Health

The critical importance of a family for the developing child is universally recognized. Family interactions of mother, father, and young child leave an indelible impression upon the child's personality. Down through the ages and across the many cultures of man, the family in some form or other has been the most durable of our social institutions. Too often the family is taken for granted because of its pervasive influence. One only has to experience a disruption of the family or the loss of a loved one to realize its fundamental importance. Families differ markedly in their lifestyle, social interaction, cohesiveness, size, and the degree to which grandparents, aunts, uncles, and others are thought of as part of the extended family.

Family patterns are changing in ways that spell trouble for the children of our society and their parents. The National Academy of Sciences published a major report by the National Research Council

(1976) aimed at establishing a new national policy for children and families. Among the disturbing statistical trends noted in this report are the following:

1. One out of every six children under the age of eighteen now lives in a family with only one parent—double the percentage of single-parent families in 1950. In single-parent families, the absent member is usually the father. The effect of father's absence depends largely upon why he is absent and the attitudes that remain after his departure. Children can develop normally in a single-parent home but such development is often difficult. Adequate alternative supervision of the child must be provided while the parent works; there must be adequate contact with the child when the parent is at home; and the absent parent should not be denigrated in the eyes of the child.

2. Adult family members are less available to children today than they were a generation ago. The number of working mothers with preschool children has tripled since 1950, while the proportion of mothers with school-age children has doubled. More children than ever are left to fend for themselves. The passive viewing of television after school hours has substituted for parent-child interaction in all too many homes.

3. The number of illegitimate births, mostly to teenage mothers, has increased sharply in the past fifteen years. Today one out of every eight births is illegitimate. About 10 percent of American teenagers get pregnant and 6 percent give birth each year.

The Alan Guttmacher Institute (1976) reported that more than half the twenty-one million teenagers in the United States are sexually active. Only 28 percent of babies conceived by the 600,000 teenagers who gave birth in 1974 followed marriage. Although fertility in general has declined since 1960, birthrates among young girls have actually risen. This epidemic of adolescent pregnancies contributes significantly to the number of infants and young children who receive inadequate care. U.S. teenage child-bearing rates are among the world's highest. The frequent lack of prenatal care and the young age of these mothers produce an unusually high percentage of babies who are underweight and frail.

4. Child abuse, infanticide, teenage suicide, school dropouts, drug use, and juvenile delinquency have increased concurrently with these other major social changes in the family. Youngsters growing up

in low-income families are at a specially high risk of damage physically, intellectually, emotionally, and socially.

5. The middle-class American family of today increasingly resembles the low-income family of the early 1960s on most of the indices of social disorder. Quite clearly, the children of so-called traditional families are also in serious trouble to a higher degree than our society can tolerate.

A child's cultural milieu and family environment have a more profound impact on mental health and illness than upon any other aspect of individual well being because of the interpersonal and behavioral nature of mental health.

Early intervention with infants and preschool children has proven promising as a preventative approach, provided certain general guidelines are carefully followed. In a review of large-scale experiments in the United States, Urie Bronfenbrenner (1974) has formulated some principles of early intervention that are worth noting. Foremost among these principles is the development of family-centered intervention. Evidence to date indicates that the family is the most effective and economical means for fostering development of the child. Active participation of family members is critical to the success of any intervention program. Ideally, intervention begins in preparation for parenthood and in providing an adequate cultural milieu for nurturing the newborn infant.

Large-scale parent-child development centers established as national experiments have clearly demonstrated the value of parental training during the child's first years of life followed by preschool group experiences in which parent and child continue to work closely together. Highly significant results have been obtained not only for disadvantaged black minorities but also for middle-class white families, Spanish-speaking Mexican-Americans, and other ethnic groups. A closer look at a representative parent-child development center for Spanish-speaking Mexican-American children in Houston, Texas, illustrates the way in which this type of educational-social intervention improves the mental health of children and their families.

In the Houston model program, social intervention consists of working closely with both the mothers and fathers of very young children. Beginning at the age of twelve months, a bilingual worker makes frequent home visits to introduce the mother to a number of techniques for intellectual stimulation of the child. The mother is coached in her communication with the child in order to promote cognitive and personality growth while maintaining strong affectional bonds with her child. Parents meet regularly several evenings a month to discuss their family problems, to share their ideas, and to seek advice. The family is dealt with as a whole and the techniques are carefully adapted to the cultural milieu in which the family lives. Consequently, the parents are uniformly enthusiastic.

When the child is two years old, mother and child attend a special nursery school four mornings a week. Parent-child relations continue to be stressed at the nursery at the same time that the child is introduced to social interactions with other children in a controlled and stimulating but playful environment. Videotape recordings of mother-child interactions are played back for the mother so that she can see where she is facilitating or inhibiting desired behavior in the child. Periodic contacts with the family are maintained after the child is three years old in preparation for the youngster's entering school.

A model program of this type incorporating all of the best techniques from earlier experiments is expensive, particularly when carried out with a great deal of accompanying research and evaluation. Most of the essentials of such a preschool program, however, can be applied without a great financial investment by use of volunteers and the heavy involvement of parents. Still, one can rightly ask whether or not the benefits from such a model program are worth the costs. The final answers to this important question are not yet available. Nevertheless, early returns from evaluative research in the Houston project indicate the following important findings when the experimental families in the program are compared to similar families who do not participate:

1. As compared to controls, the program mothers grew significantly more affectionate, encouraged more child verbalization, showed more praise, and had children who were more verbally responsive.

2. Home observation scales revealed greater maternal involvement with the child, greater emotional and verbal responsiveness of the mother, avoidance of restriction and punishment, and more provision of appropriate play materials on the part of the program mothers.

3. Children in the experiment maintained a nearly constant level of mental ability over time, as measured by the Bayley Scales and

Stanford-Binet, while the control children fell steadily behind the norm.

A grant from the Hogg Foundation for Mental Health (an endowment within The University of Texas System, which functions as a granting foundation to support demonstration projects in mental health) to the University of Houston has made possible a follow-up study of both experimental and control children in the Houston Parent-Child Development Center in order to determine the extent to which these early experiences and parental training have an ongoing helpful influence upon the child's later mental and emotional development. Results indicate that the program does indeed have lasting effects of a positive nature. The elegant simplicity of this parent-child development center approach takes advantage of informal support systems and is readily adaptable to other ethnic and cultural groups.

Cultural and Social Change

A second and often underplayed factor in understanding mental health components influencing people today is the alteration of societal makeup. Acceptable family patterns and child-rearing practices undergo continuous refinement as society changes. Transmitting the primary values, skills, and other personality characteristics from one generation to the next is the key to survival as a society. Granted that biological as well as social factors enter into the development of an individual personality, certain shared attitudes, beliefs, and values within the culture provide a common basis for socialization of the child.

These implicit attitudes, beliefs, and values constitute sociocultural premises that are fundamental determinants of shared personality characteristics within a given culture. For these reasons, studies of families and their children within different cultures can shed considerable light upon the significance of both psychological and cultural factors as they influence the mental health and development of the individual.

A six-year longitudinal study of more than 800 children and their families in Mexico and the United States illustrates the importance of cultural factors in child development (Holtzman et al, 1975). A large staff of research associates in Mexico City and Austin, Texas, gave an extensive battery of psychological tests to each child once a year for six years. The children were originally drawn from the first, fourth, and seventh grades so that a complete developmental continuum from age six to seventeen could be covered in the six years of repeated testing.

Pairs of cases were closely matched across the two cultures in order to control for socioeconomic status, age, and sex of the child. Midway through the study, intensive interviews were conducted with the mothers in their homes in order to obtain information about the family lifestyle, home environment, parental aspirations for the child, child-rearing practices, and other factors believed to be important influences upon the child's development.

Most of the differences in personality discovered between Mexican and Anglo-American children can be attributed to the differing sociocultural premises underlying the two cultures. The majority of adolescent Americans subscribe to active self-assertion as a sociocultural premise while their Mexican counterparts prefer affiliative obedience. Mexicans tend to be more family-centered and cooperative in interpersonal activities while Americans are more individual-centered and competitive.

Similar findings concerning the importance of informal social support systems in sustaining an individual's mental health have been reported by Gary (1979) in promoting mental health in black communities. Focusing on the strengths of black people and the positive aspects of their mental health, Gary and his colleagues singled out the black churches and the extended family network as vital social support systems that have been ignored too long by professional mental health workers.

Hispanic Culture

The fastest growing minority population in the United States consists of Hispanic Americans, particularly those of Mexican descent. Competition, ethnocentrism, and conflict among the ethnic populations of the Southwest have taken their toll upon the Mexican-American for more than a century. One would expect that as a result of the stresses and frustrations suffered by the Mexican-American, a greater incidence of mental illness and severe emotional disturbances would be present among the Mexican-Americans than among the Anglos. The first systematic data collected on this important question were gathered over twenty-five years ago by E. Gartley Jaco in a major study supported by the Hogg Foundation. Jaco surveyed all inhabitants of the state of Texas who sought psychiatric treatment for a psychosis for the first time in their lives during the two-year period of 1951–1952 (Jaco, 1959). Information was compiled from every psychiatrist in private practice as well as from all the hospitals and clinics in Texas and surrounding states.

The results showed only 6 percent of the new psychotic cases during this two-year period were Mexican-American; 85 percent were Anglo-Americans; and the remainder were primarily black. When the data were standardized for age and sex composition, the average annual incidence rate per 100,000 population was only 42 for the Mexican-Americans. The same incidence rate for Anglos was 80, while that for blacks was 56.

Additional checking by Jaco convinced him that the markedly lower incidence rate for psychosis among Mexican-Americans was not a function of accessibility of treatment. Could the lower incidence rate for Mexican-Americans result from different ways of coping with stress? Could the smaller number be due to more cohesive family patterns and different lifestyles? Or is the rate, at least in part, only illusory because the Mexican-American seeks out *curanderos* rather than psychiatrists when mental illness is present?

In 1957 with Hogg Foundation support, William Madsen, Antonieta Espejo, Octavio Romano, and Arthur Rubel embarked upon a three-year anthropological project dealing with differential culture change and mental health in south Texas (Rubel, 1966). After intensive ethnographic studies of three variations of Mexican-American folk culture in which the referral networks for curing illness were carefully traced, Madsen and his colleagues concluded that the different world views and ways of coping with illness that characterized the Mexican folk culture and urban Anglo society are sufficient to account for a large part of Jaco's findings.

Madsen proposed that stress situations among Mexican-Americans are less likely to produce mental illness because they are shared by the family group (Madsen, 1969). He hypothesized that anxiety-producing stress seldom precipitates mental illness when the anxiety is shared and relieved by a tightly knit, primary group like the Mexican family.

Later studies by M. Karno and R. B. Edgerton (1969) indicate that mental illness is also greatly underrepresented among the Mexican-Americans of Los Angeles, a large metropolitan population rather far removed from the folk culture of rural south Texas. Edgerton found that folk-psychiatry had greatly diminished in influence among Los Angeles Mexican-Americans and that the great majority of Mexican-Americans would not hesitate to seek help from a psychiatrist or mental health clinic (Edgerton, Karno, Fernandez, 1970), a finding confirmed more recently by J. M. Casas, S. E. Keefe, A. Padilla, and others (1978) at the Spanish Speaking Mental Health Research Center in Los Angeles.

Whatever the reasons for the lower incidence of mental illness among Mexican-Americans, it is clear that recognition of mental illness is a social process. Rather than a problem in medical diagnosis, the recognition of mental illness is a social transaction that often takes the form of a negotiation. The symptomatic content and prevalence of mental illness in various populations are dependent to a large extent upon how this negotiable social transaction is carried out.

Specific Needs

Severe mental illnesses such as schizophrenia or depressive psychoses are only one aspect of mental health problems requiring community services tailored to specific cultures. Chronic alcoholism, drug addiction, social alienation, child abuse, crime and delinquency, some forms of interpersonal aggression, dehumanizing and degrading social practices, family disintegration, neurotic behavior, and a host of other common psychological and social problems are of even greater importance in a society that is searching for better ways to promote mental and emotional health for all of its people.

Absence of mental illness is not synonymous with the presence of mental health. Everyone is faced at some time in life with identity crises, severe emotional stress, frustration, and failure. At one time or another each person desperately needs help. A mentally healthy person is not only one who has learned to cope with most life stresses but also one who understands when help is needed.

While every culture has some way of coping with psychological and social problems, complex industrialized societies create for their members unusual stresses that require professionally trained persons to provide a wide range of services to people in need of help. For each highly trained professional in the mental health field a team of para-professionals, technicians, and volunteer workers is needed in order for services to be effective. A major problem for the disadvantaged and culturally different has been the severe lack of adequately trained personnel indigenous to the people served. Most professionals come from middle-class Anglo-American backgrounds, creating acute shortages of service delivery personnel who can be most effective for the large number of relatively uneducated, lower-class families who desperately need help.

Since global services always translate into personal ones, some of the historical developments and specific concerns may be traced with examples from the vantage point of one organization.

Texas and the Hogg Foundation for Mental Health

Unlike the older states of the Midwest and East, Texas has only recently become a predominantly urban society with both the opportunities and problems characteristic of large cities. Thirty years ago few psychiatrists and almost no psychologists or psychiatric social workers practiced in public service. A major state hospital boasted of only one board-certified psychiatrist for several thousand patients. Ancient buildings and archaic practices characterized the state hospitals, and almost no public out-patient facilities were available.

The newly established Hogg Foundation for Mental Hygiene, made possible by the estate of Will Hogg and the wisdom of his surviving sister, Ima, offered hope for significant change. Miss Hogg had gained her early understanding of emotional needs and social problems from her father, Governor James Stephen Hogg. Robert L. Sutherland, a sociologist who served at the first director of the Hogg Foundation, devoted his energies in the early years to educating the people of

Texas about mental health. From its beginning, the Hogg Foundation adopted a pluralistic concept of mental health encompassing social and cultural factors as well as psychological and medical concerns in its program of public education, consultation, and support of mental health programs throughout the state.

By 1954 the income of the Foundation doubled, making possible the launching of new programs. Additional emphasis was given to research in the social and behavioral sciences where there were promising young investigators whose reputations were not sufficiently well-established to interest sources of federal grants. Investment of only $80,000 of private funds by the Hogg Foundation was largely responsible for attracting more than $1 million in grants over the next three years. A number of these projects were aimed at gaining a better understanding of how to provide more effective mental health services for Mexican-Americans, blacks, small-town residents, and the rural poor, as well as inner city dwellers. An increased concern for the underlying problems of society characterized the Foundation's work in the 1960s.

The major thrust of the Hogg Foundation has shifted from one emphasis to another, with each change dictated by the critical needs and opportunities of the time. In 1963 Texas received its first planning grant from the federal government to develop a comprehensive mental health plan for the entire state. Officers of the Hogg Foundation joined with other citizens in a number of task forces appointed by the governor, from which a new Texas Department of Mental Health and Mental Retardation emerged two years later. Within the first three years of the new department's operation, twenty-four community mental health and mental retardation centers were established. In addition, the state hospitals began an outreach network that provided public services in areas beyond the bounds of the new mental health centers. With this shift of emphasis to local services, the resident population of state mental hospitals dropped to one-third over the following thirteen years. At the same time, appropriations for the community services rose from $600,000 to over $41 million. In spite of this progress, however, many citizens throughout the state strongly believed that further changes were urgently needed in order to provide more effective services for all the people of Texas.

Sensing an opportunity to bring many organizations and leaders together in a new reform movement, the Hogg Foundation organized the first Robert Lee Sutherland Seminar on Mental Health as a tribute to its late president in May 1978. The central theme of the conference, "Mental Health for the People of Texas," used the just-published report of the President's Commission on Mental Health as a catalyst to bring together nearly a thousand citizens from all areas of life. Out of the workshops, lectures, and seminars highlighted by Rosalynn Carter's keynote address, a new organization was launched—Citizens for Human Development. To carry out a massive public education program funded by private as well as public monies, this citizens' movement is aimed at new legislation and greatly increased support at the local level for community mental health services (DeMoll & Andrade, 1978).

Both private and public funds are seen as essential to the success of mental health services at the community level. While the principal source of funds must remain public appropriations from the federal and state levels, delivery of human services will prove truly effective only if private and local funds are assured, together with the enthusiastic voluntary contributions of local citizens. The American tradition of private giving for public purposes preserves the essential elements of freedom and flexibility that are critical for local success. How all the needs of a community relate to one another and ways to define the nature of mental health services in terms of local tradition, local resources, and local motivations are beyond the reach of both federal and state governments. The nonprofit private sector of our society has a vital role to play in the seeking of new solutions to human problems at the local level. As John Gardner, former Secretary of Health, Education, and Welfare and founder of Common Cause, has stated in the creation of a new organization aimed at strengthening the private pursuit of public purpose, "Thanks to the institutions of the non-profit sector, not only can citizens participate in the concerns of American life, they can do so at the grass roots level— and in doing so contribute importantly to the preservation of vital communities" (1979).

Among the most important aspects of our communities that are an essential part of a healthy private sector is the web of personal, familial, and neighborly relations. These ties are essential as informal support systems in the resolution of family and personal crises. All too frequently the categorical funding and federal or state regulations accompanying mental health service programs lead to tragic disruption, rather than facilitation, of these indigenous forces at the local level.

The Hogg Foundation for Mental Health is but one small illustration of a privately endowed organization striving to nourish the indigenous resources latent in all of our communities. While only a tiny number of the 26,000 private foundations in the United States have mental health as a specific focus, many are concerned with more effective human services at the local level. Churches, the United Way, civic clubs, and other private organizations are equally concerned with the preservation of the informal support systems that can restore our sense of community. Citizen participation at the grass roots level clearly provides the best opportunity for sympathetic personal attention to human problems.

Summary

In this presentation of some ideas concerning social and cultural influences upon the delivery of mental health services, a few key points can be highlighted. The report of the President's Commission on Mental Health and other recent studies all indicate an urgent need for strengthening the grass roots involvement of local citizens in the development of more effective mental health services. A focus upon the underserved and the sociocultural factors that must be taken into account has been neglected too long in our efforts to mount large comprehensive systems of mental health.

Important issues can be summarized in a set of principles, as follows:

First, the definition of mental illness is a social contract subject to wide variations of interpretation depending upon the cultural context and social norms of the community.

Second, the degree to which services are used is directly related to their accessibility and appropriateness as defined in sociocultural terms by the individuals constituting the community.

Third, indigenous systems of support, both social and family, are hidden assets that must be recognized and strengthened rather than thoughtlessly destroyed.

Fourth, the farther removed the sources of funding and control from the community being served, the more unresponsive and irrelevant is the agency's response to community needs is likely to be.

And finally, it must be remembered that the organization and delivery of services from the consumers' point of view is often markedly different from the viewpoint of the service providers.

The community mental health center movement is at a crossroad where it can either recede back into more traditional, narrowly defined psychiatric services closely associated with mental hospitals, or it can go through further transformation in becoming a more responsive, highly flexible system of services under local control and direction. Whether or not the new Mental Health Systems Act can accomplish this transformation remains to be seen. That plan has its strongest chances to succeed if everyone within the community mental health movement takes seriously the major issues raised.

References

Alan Guttmacher Institute. *11 Million Teenagers: What Can Be Done About the Epidemic of Adolescent Pregnancies in the United States.* New York: Planned Parenthood Federation of America, 1976.

Bronfenbrenner, U. *A Report on Longitudinal Evaluations of Preschool Programs: Is Early Intervention Effective?*, vol. 2. Washington, D.C.: Department of Health, Education, and Welfare, publication number (OHD) 74-25, 1974.

Brown, B. From custody to compassion—Brown cites strides of NIMH. *Psychiatric News* (August 15, 1973), p. 11.

Casas, J. M., & Keefe, S. E. (eds.). *Family and Mental Health in the Mexican American Community.* Los Angeles: University of California Spanish Speaking Mental Health Research Center, 1978.

DeMoll, L. E., & Andrade, S. J. (eds.). *Mental Health for the People of Texas.* Austin: Hogg Foundation for Mental Health, 1978.

Edgerton, R. B., Karno, M., & Fernandez, I. Curanderismo in the metropolis: The diminishing role of folk-psychiatry among Los Angeles Mexican-Americans. *American Journal of Psychotherapy* 24: 124–134, 1970.

Gardner, J. The private pursuit of public purpose. *The Chronicle of Higher Education* (January 8, 1979).

Gary, L. E. (ed.) *Mental Health: A Challenge to Black Community*. Ardmore, Penn.: Dorrance & Company, 1979.

Holtzman, W. H., Diaz-Guerrero, R., & Swartz, J. D. *Personality Development in Two Cultures*. Austin: University of Texas Press, 1975.

Jaco, E. G. Mental Health of the Spanish-American in Texas. In M. K. Opler, Ed., *Culture and Mental Health*. New York: Macmillan Company, 1959, pp. 467–485.

Karno, M., & Edgerton, R. B. Perception of mental illness in a Mexican-American community. *Archives of General Psychiatry* 20: 223–238, 1969.

Klerman, G. L. Mental Illness, the medical model, and psychiatry. *The Journal of Medicine and Philosophy* 2: 220–243, 1977.

Madsen, W. Mexican-Americans and Anglo-Americans: A comparative study of mental health in Texas. In S. C. Plog, & R. B. Edgerton (eds.). *Changing Perspectives in Mental Illness*. New York: Holt, Rinehart, & Winston, 1969, pp. 217–241.

National Research Council. *Toward a National Policy for Children and Families*. Advisory Committee on Child Development. Washington, D.C.: National Academy of Sciences, 1976.

President's Commission on Mental Health. *Report to the President from the President's Commission on Mental Health*. Washington, D.C.: U.S. Government Printing Office, 1978.

Rubel, A. *Across the Tracks: Mexican-Americans in a Texas City*. Austin: The University of Texas, 1966.

Optimum Clinical Environment?
Is This the Way?

N. Archer Moore, Ph.D.

The optimum clinical environment is the optimum environment for which a healthy change can be effected in individuals so desiring to change, or, for that matter, in individuals for whom others have determined a change is necessary. Certainly, the optimum environment is probably beyond our abilities to define, given the state of the art of psychotherapy today. Certainly, no particular school of thought has been notably more successful than any other, although individuals within several schools of thought seem to have amassed a better-than-average batting average.

To some extent the limelight of psychotherapy, and the clinical environment along with it, has been left to the work of some of our more charismatic personalities. The difficulty with the charismatic personality is not just that he/she may be selling self rather than salvation, but that he/she tends sooner or later to invoke a number of followers or disciples. Unfortunately, most disciples tend to apply the "teachings" verbatim to all problems presented rather than to evolve better approaches.

In spite of the fact that no particular school of thought seems to have the answer, all of them are rather busily propagating the answers that they do have. As evidence of this propagation I am sure all you have to do is collect "workshop literature" in your mail for a few months' time. This new trend seems to be an attempt to exploit continuing education legislation recently enacted.

At this time I certainly do not feel that we can define anything like an optimum environment for treating the emotional difficulties of the population. However, the recent upsurges in quasi-religious sects certainly indicate that the number of problems that need treatment have not lessened. These quasi-religions almost without fail talk more about emotional peace of mind than life in the hereafter. It is as though a certain portion of the ministry has given up on the concept of sin and substituted salvation from emotional ills instead.

Even among the more professionally treatment-oriented mental health disciples we find a fantastic array of alternate systems. We have bio-energetics to energize us and primal screams to awaken us. We have TA to help us find the child in ourselves and Behavior Mod if we don't like him once found. We can elect to follow the chants of the Arica Foundation or meditate transcendentally. We can engage in Gestalt awareness, attend a "stroke-a-thon," or chart our way through all these mystifying realms by psychic astrology. In the event that we feel in danger of losing our mental grip on things, we can seek the services of one of the Silva Mind Control groups. On the other hand, if we seem not to be getting the most out of things, we may train our sensitivity to body massages and become accustomed to "eating what comes naturally." If all else fails, we can enroll in assertiveness training for women, blacks, gays, marijuana users, etc. If we accidentally become parents, courses to improve our parenting abilities rival the federal government in finding catchy letter symbols from Stepping to Petting.

It occurs to me that each approach listed in our program, be it hospital, university, private practice, natural environment, or self-help, offers adequate solutions to certain types of problems but certainly not to all. In spite of the fact that there has been a move to depopulate our hospitals, I find that we have, in effect, substituted a revolving system that rotates the same patient population on a merry-go-round beginning with the community outpatient center, the emergency room, or local receiving ward of the city hospital and returning to the psychiatric hospital. Thus, while people are being revolved in and out of the hospital it appears to me that little is done toward making them either more useful or more happy citizens.

Also, the involved paper problems of these procedures have become staggering. In some centers the clerical staff outnumbers the professional workers. Indeed, we are in danger of becoming experts in treating paper rather than people.

Universities that maintain treatment centers are primarily interested in young practitioners. These universities have an opportunity to offer the latest techniques of the hospital as well as research capacities. One should normally expect that more progress would come from such an environment. However, the fault here is that most universities tend to treat a population with better-than-average intelligence who are not especially economically or culturally deprived. Thus, treatment regimens that work well with college-educated people do not necessarily fit the needs of the inner city, or the outer country, for that matter.

The limitation of private practices is that they simply cannot afford to deal with the grosser emotional problems. Unfortunately, even when government programs are enacted to underwrite a portion, and, I emphasize a portion, of the expense of treating the economically deprived, these programs usually are handled with such cumbersome bureaucratic procedures that the patient frequently is denied access to most of the experienced private practitioners. In addition, artificial limits are usually placed on the length of treatment on economic grounds rather than on the need of the patient.

I am not sure that I am adequate to deal with natural environment since I feel that it is our natural (or perhaps unnatural) environment that has produced the problem. Certainly, in private practice one does little to remove the subject from the natural environment, although we might at times heartily wish that we could.

Self-help has received much publicity. In an address at a seminar at the University of Hawaii their Dean of Public Health, Gerald M. Michael, pointed out that most human ills are closely associated with behavioral patterns. He cited as population ills everything from arthritis and rheumatism to malignant neoplasms and suicide. He indicated that the individual's own habits, such as cigarette smoking and excessive psychological stress, predisposes the organism to these various ills. In spite of our excellent educational system, little behavioral change seems to have been effected, whether we utilize modern advertising on television or more traditional educational approaches in our university centers and our public schools.

People who suffer from emotional illnesses are seldom in need of education. It is at this point that the distinction needs to be drawn between the counselor's skills and the therapist. A number of people counsel and do so quite well—teachers, lawyers, ministers, family physicians, parents—to name but a few. The problem with the emotionally ill person is not the lack of counseling in what is appropriate behavior; too often the patient persists in exhibiting inappropriate behavior in spite of the counseling. When we deal with the problem of why a particular individual persists in self-destructive behavioral mechanisms in the face of logic and education, we are dealing with therapy. To function adequately as a psychotherapist one must be acutely aware of when to function as a counselor and when to function as a therapist.

It is my own personal opinion that self-help literature is entertaining but likely to be ineffective in terms of actually changing lifestyles. This puts me in a rather uncomfortable position of criticizing the many volumes that abound in today's market, yet the ideas espoused by most of them are quite sound. I certainly would not want the public in general to ignore practicing good emotional health any more than I would want them to cease practicing good oral hygiene. However, since the practice of oral hygiene alone does not make one a dentist, I do not think the reading of countless "how to improve" books makes one necessarily the best therapist.

In my opinion, the best help is that which helps the least. In other words, a patient can quickly become overwhelmed and made to feel manipulated into health by either modifying behavior or injecting a certain number of foreign chemicals into the body. As useful as these are, they usually entail engendering some form of dependence. Thus, in my private practice I tend to attempt to gain the cooperation of the person with the problem so that he/she begins not only to understand the problem but also to take some responsibility for the problem.

Of course, this discussion is not to belittle the role of the therapist, which I tend to take as more than an impartial or objective observer. The therapist, in order to treat, must be willing not only to understand that the other person is suffering but also to share some of that suffering. I continually remind myself that progress in psychotherapy is usually slow and often painful. However, if a therapist expects to share in the exhilaration of the "Ah ha!" insights and breakthroughs, he/she must also share in frustrations of the "Oh Sh——!" experience.

From my vantage point as a private practitioner as well as a consultant to several agencies, I am convinced that most successful treatment takes training, experience, and dedication. All of these conditions are necessary and none are sufficient without the others. I think that it is high time that we professionals in the mental health area state in no uncertain terms that there are no shortcuts to emotional maturity and that personal health and happiness is a life/growth process that is either improving or getting worse but seldom standing still. If begun early enough and tended with care it can be found by most, but not without real dedication.

Community-based Treatment as an Optimum Clinical Environment

Ruth Ann Lyman, Ph.D.

In any consideration of the various clinical environments and their respective unique strengths, the community-based alternative must assume its logical position as a viable, effective treatment environment. It is the treatment environment of choice for many clients and practitioners and on that basis alone may be viewed as an optimum clinical environment. But in addition to the benefits, strictly clinical and otherwise, for the client, his/her family, and the practitioner, community-based treatment reflects a broad range of positive features typically minimized in assessing the pros and cons of a clinical setting. These features involve issues concerning and affecting the community at large, or the local public, and governmental participants in the financial support of both private and public systems of mental health care. Overall, the community-based alternative may be considered the optimum clinical environment recognizing its clinical treatment potential as well as its advantageous social and economic facets.

Before enumerating these factors, however, three points of clarification should be stressed. First, the descriptor "optimum clinical environment" escapes precise definition. It is used within this context to mean an external environment, usually in which treatment takes place, which best contributes to, enhances, or facilitates treatment and the lasting effects of treatment. The particular topic at hand is the community-based treatment environment and refers to the setting in which an individual receives treatment services within his or her local community. Data suggest that treatment within this environment is usually on an outpatient basis; but treatment within the community environment may include functionally a broad range of treatment modalities such as residential care, partial hospitalization, short-term hospitalization, and other specialized services for particular populations, including the alcoholic and drug abuser. This expanded range of services is commonly available through community mental health centers or other clinics and treatment facilities operating under private or public sponsorship. Conceptually, many of the particular benefits that may be derived via the community-based treatment approach are consistent with the individual or group private practice model for psychiatrists, psychologists, and other mental health professionals. Basically, community-based treatment is most dramatically contrasted with the institutional environment.

The second point of clarification involves the changing definition of optimum clinical environment as a function of individual patient needs. To promote one clinical environment as the optimum clinical environment would be presumptuous, given the present state of the art of psychotherapy. The true optimum clinical environment will vary from individual to individual, perhaps even from time to time and circumstance to circumstance. No one clinical environment can be optimum for every client in need of treatment. Therefore, from a client viewpoint, there is no one optimum clinical environment, and on the whole an optimum clinical environment cannot be defined or determined on a group basis.

Third, from the outset it must be emphasized that the unique positive features of community-based treatment are completely contingent upon the appropriate application of this approach. For example, in the case of a patient requiring long-term hospitalization or a more restrictive environment than available in the community, this option would be far from optimum; treatment within the community environment when not appropriate would at best invalidate the factors presented herein. Having recognized the requisite of proper application, community-based treatment can be presented as an optimum clinical environment, the alternative of choice from a variety of perspectives.

Factors that contribute to the community approach generally fall into five categories: clinical treatment factors, quasi-clinical client factors, community factors, governmental and economic issues, and staff/practitioner factors. The clinical treatment and client factors must function as the most powerful and stringent criteria in considering a setting as optimum, for treatment is the fundamental purpose of the therapist's endeavor.

Two of the clearest clinical advantages to the community-based treatment approach involve the use of natural support systems and the maintenance of exposure to a functional model. Treatment carried out in the client's "home ground" provides better access to family, friends, teachers, and other members of the client's natural interpersonal environment who may function as natural support systems. Family members, for example, can more readily participate in the treatment process as appropriate. Equally important, community-based treatment does not require isolation from support systems, whereas institutional-based treatment may require an arbitrary or artificial division between the client and such systems, oftentimes when the system can be helpful to the client and the treatment process. Indirectly, community-based treatment may foster more acceptance and understanding of the emotional/psychological disorders, family and related systems' investment in progress rather than illness, and improved education concerning factors involved in mental illness and its treatment. Globally, a long-range outcome might be a more enlightened community and a weakening of the still powerful stigma borne by most who seek "mental treatment."

Clients treated within the community are also presented with a functional model as opposed to a disfunctional model that prevails within most institutional and long-term care facilities. Exposure to the functional model may facilitate clearer and more direct feedback to the client concerning societal expectations, behavioral consequences, and real-world contingencies, both in a strict "treatment" sense and in the client's day-to-day operations.

For most clients, the "criterion environment" in which one seeks to survive and succeed is the broad community environment, not within an isolated, protected environment or institution. Therefore, psychotherapeutic progress effected in the community or on the "home ground" facilitates generalization to the client's usual living situation. Barriers to effective generalization of treatment gains have remained substantial handicaps of institutional treatment. With due respect to the particular advantages of these treatment settings, problems of generalizing treatment gains are minimized when gains are achieved in an environment more closely resembling "the criterion environment." This reduction of barriers may be viewed as a significant clinical advantage to community-based treatment.

Continuity of care is a fourth benefit for the client and his/her treatment process, as well as a benefit for the therapist. The therapist can follow the client from treatment modality to modality if necessary, such as from hospitalization to partial care, or from residential half-way house to outpatient treatment. This continuity is particularly apparent within community mental health center settings.

Perhaps the benefit that applies across the board to clinical issues, client factors, community matters, and even social and economic aspects, is the opportunity for the client's continued productivity. In most cases, there is no need for physical relocation, even in the event that a short period of hospitalization is advisable. Many clients treated within the community can stay on the job, maintain an income, continue in school, remain with family, interact socially, and generally function to some degree as a contributing and active member of society. Clearly, the client profits in many ways, while the community profits as well through the client's social, economic, and civic productivity concomitant with the treatment process. In addition, the fact of maintaining such productivity may further weaken the stigma associated with mental illness.

Aside from clinical, client-oriented, and family-related aspects, economic matters must be assessed. Budget comparisons with institutional treatment demonstrate the cost effectiveness of the community-based system. Coupled with the social and economic benefits to the client, family, and community mentioned earlier, the community environment presents powerful, positive economic features to a number of publics. Cost effectiveness and its potential for cost control appeal to governmental participants in the funding of mental health care programs; considering today's overall economic atmosphere, this issue is certainly powerful and timely. Without detailing the complex matrix of factors influencing cost considerations, one may observe that given the appropriateness of community-based treatment, it is one of the more cost-effective approaches. Dollars are expended almost exclusively on treatment services without involving large expenditures for food, housing, transportation, and other living expenses for large numbers of clients. It should also be recognized that a factor with economic and treatment implications is the potential for utilizing "natural" therapists (family, teachers, coaches, ministers, and so forth) as opposed to the almost exclusive use of expensive medical and mental health professional and paraprofessional staff in institutional settings.

As a result of many of these types of factors, an overall benefit to the community and to the potential client is increased visibility of the problems and current concerns of the mentally ill. Visibility within this context refers to the issue conceptually and generally, rather than to visibility of individuals diagnosed as mentally ill or in treatment. Effects may include higher potential for community awareness, and indeed involvement or support in such issues. Perhaps such visibility will help weaken the stigma associated with mental illness. It is even possible such visibility could stimulate improved support for preventive and mental health education programs on a local level.

The strength of community-based mental health services have focused exclusively on the client, the family, and the community. To complete this review of community-based treatment as an optimum clinical environment, the positive potential for mental health practitioners must at least be briefly mentioned.

One of the clearest attractions for most therapists is the opportunity to work with a variety of clients, particularly in terms of levels of functioning. The therapist may work with clients having severe psychotic symptoms or with those showing minor behavior problems, with the chronic alcoholic or with families exhibiting chronic patterns of pathology. There may be the additional opportunity for participation in patient education programs. In such a setting, the norms of the mental health practitioner may be maintained somewhat better than long-term employment in an institutional setting.

A second advantage the mental health practitioner identifies is the direct or indirect knowledge that enables the therapist to judge progress against criterion environment. Such knowledge has direct implications for quality or treatment concerns as well.

A third point is the stimulation of the interdisciplinary staff. Community-based treatment appears to provide better opportunity for interdisciplinary contact and learning, regular consultation and input across disciplinary lines, and more flexibility with treatment models than in settings that employ only the medical model.

The final advantage of community-based treatment for the clinical practitioner is a multifaceted feature that benefits client, community, and therapist alike. This factor is community systems awareness. Community mental health center staffs or practitioners in similar programs are aware of a wide range of helping agencies (such as Legal Aide, Vocational Rehabilitation Services, Department of Pensions and Security, Sheltered Workshops) to which clients and families can be referred. Also, staff may be in a position to perform a case management function that assists in assuring appropriate utilization of human service agencies, plus follow-through in the use of those services. Additionally, community systems can be used concurrently rather than being artificially linked by time as other settings may require. For example, a client may be treated through a residential facility while at the same time receiving service through a vocational rehabilitation system; a client enrolled in a day treatment program may also profit from legal aid services and welfare services at the same time.

Although no one clinical environment may be considered optimum in all treatment cases, the community-based environment offers many individual strengths and advantages. The community-based system enhances clinical treatment and provides quasi-clinical benefits to client, family, and staff. The community and the public funders of health care systems also realize social and economic benefits especially in comparison to the more traditional institutional approaches to treatment.

Concerns and Issues Involving a Board of Directors and Its Relationship to Staff

James W. Fryer, B.S. Ind. Mgmt.

The board approach to management presents certain problems, inherent in the method itself, for public and private organizations. It has been observed that such (inherent) problems become very limiting to organizational effectiveness and efficiency when available measures are not employed to reduce ambiguity, uncertainty, and confusion as to management roles and responsibilities. Observations and recommendations regarding board problems and concerns in organizing and operating community centers are herein presented which, if adequately implemented, give reason for optimism regarding board governance of Texas Mental Health and Mental Retardation (MHMR) centers.

Staff in Texas community centers range in size from less than 40 to more than 600 persons. Trustees are appointed by city and county governments, school districts, and hospital districts, or various combinations of all of these. Because centers serve varying demographic and geographic constituencies, board and staff operational problems and concerns are in great contrast. The situations in Houston (Harris County) and Amarillo are examples: the Harris County center serves a large, dense population with few service contracts and one appointing authority: serving twenty-one counties, most of which are sparsely settled, Amarillo has several service contracts, and more than thirty appointing authorities.

Observations—Community Centers

Board Responsibilities and Characteristics

In Texas, "the board of trustees is responsible for the administration

94

of community centers";[1] boards are required to appoint a director (usually termed an executive director) and *may* delegate the administration to the executive director.

Professional people such as attorneys, accountants, educators, and persons in public life and banking constitute the majority of the Texas board members. A few are engineers, ranchers, farmers, homemakers, dentists, or physicians. Persons experienced in higher management of organizations employing 500 or more persons are almost nonexistent among trustees.

Boards' Major Concerns

The review of Texas MHMR center operations over the past three years has revealed the following concerns as those most frequently cited by trustees to be the most significant and troublesome: community relations, client satisfaction, funding sources and management, staff morale and turnover, adequate facilities, too few competent and interested trustees, and relationships with appointing authorities.

The degree to which a board should make administrative decisions, in contrast to functioning primarily as a policy-making/performance-review body, was often in doubt. A few board members expressed uncertainty regarding key staffs' consistent adherence to approved policy.

An underlying reason for such management problems in Texas centers, readily admitted by trustees themselves, was that certain centers had not fully developed (at the time of their management audits) their board organization, board training, defined policies, planning practices, and formalized management methods. Under the circumstances community MHMR center boards have performed quite creditably. This success is attributable to the personal leadership and industry of a few key individuals appointed to most boards. However, the following quotations from over thirty past management audit reports are all too typical:

"The board had not maintained a comprehensive planning function or plan . . . (re:) long-range needs, goals, and target populations to be served . . ."

"The board had not yet implemented a program of orientation and continuing education for its members . . ."

"The board was not utilizing standing committees . . . with duties clearly defined . . ."

"The board and executive management . . . routinely submitted . . . reports that did not compare actual . . . performance . . . to planned performance."

"The board had not reported annually to sponsoring agencies and others . . . noting progress made . . ."

Boards of community centers often have had additional significant problems or needs, such as:

1. By laws inadequately providing for board operations and governance.

2. Incomplete or inadequate policies that fail to guide staff effectively and efficiently.

3. Members insufficiently committed to endure the frustrations and work load involved.

4. Members inexperienced in management processes.

5. Frustrations among members and staff in dealing with multiple funding sources and controlling agencies.

The number and nature of community center problem areas are such that it is remarkable so many boards, so much of the time, have the maximum complement of nine members.

Management Fundamentals

The fundamental processes of successful management have been generally well defined: planning, organizing, motivating, and controlling. As in most human endeavors, the statement of the principle is much simpler than the day-to-day practice. In such a nonlinear situation, the relationships have been depicted in Figure 1.[2]

The motivation and leadership aspects of management will not be fully developed here, but it is acknowledged that board and staff attitudes are obviously critical in achieving center objectives. Indeed, motivation is the "fuel" for any organizational "vehicle."

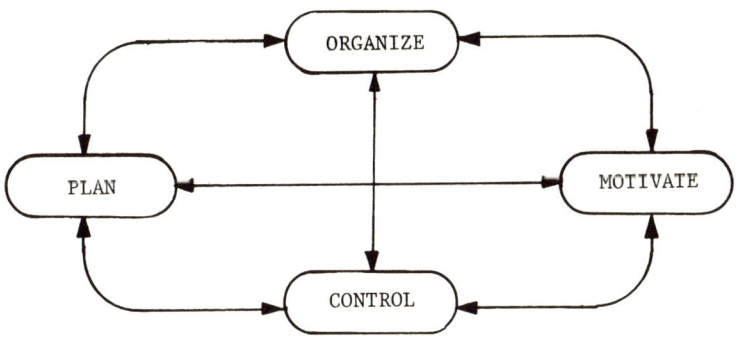

Figure 1

Board Organization

The boards of soundly managed community centers have been organized for effectiveness and efficiency by the utilization of standing (working) committees of trustees, with well-defined responsibilities and agendas. By this means a clear and well-understood division of the board's workload is achieved. Preferably, members are assigned according to interest and competence (the two are usually in consonance).

Bylaws are basic to boards' continuing effectiveness. This document should define boards' source(s) of authority, fundamental purposes and legal constraints, the officers and terms of office, board structure and standards of conduct for members, conduct of meetings, and other matters important to a clear definition of operating principles and practices.

Published policies of the board should reflect the philosophy of operation and define top-level goals or objectives, without which centers lack clear-cut guides for planning, action, and performance measurement. In addition, the responsibilities of the chief executive are defined, along with the organizational structure and programmatic roles of the entire staff.

How are the responsibilities of board and staff best divided? Robert N. Anthony effectively differentiates between top-level control and operational control in his volume *Planning and Control*.[3] Table 1 is adapted from Anthony's explanation of the two major organizational control levels.

Boards that have retained a chief executive and supporting staff capable of accepting operational responsibilities, and discharging them effectively, may safely deal almost entirely with "board control" areas such as long-range planning, organizational and operational

Table 1
Distinctions between Board-Level Control
and Operational Control

Board-Level Control	*Operational Control*
Requires concentration on a flowing, changing stream of events (often external) and needed decisions.	Concerns finite transactions and specific tasks or events.
Subjective in nature.	Essentially objective.
Judgmental decisions required, without having all information or even the variables involved.	Decision rules can be stated with all variables understood—at least conceptually.
Persuasive capability and sociopsychological awareness required.	Policies or directives usually can be followed specifically; economics or physical sciences can largely govern.
Time factors are in weeks, months, years.	Time horizon is immediate, usually day-to-day.

policies, and performance review and control, including retaining and discharging top-level staff.

Planning Performance

The planning of accomplishments, not activities, is the foundation of organizational and personal achievement. Consideration of the means, roles, and resources available is, of course, essential and may require adjustments or even curtailment of planned accomplishments for pragmatic reasons. A well-stated plan, however subject to revision, removes uncertainties and promotes the team approach to management. The goal-oriented approach to planning must be rooted in carefully enunciated top-level (board) purposes and objectives.

Controlling Operations and Resources

The control function is essential in order to assure that the organization achieves its specific objectives and therefore its broad purposes. The operations control aspect of management has been stated to comprise the following:
1. Specification of objectives.
2. Measurement of results.
3. Comparison of performance with objectives.
4. Analysis of causes of variation.
5. Determination of appropriate action.
6. Implementation of agreed actions.
7. Reappraisal and continuing adjustments.
The process must be applied at all levels of an organization.

Admittedly, there is overlap among the definitions of planning, organizing, and controlling. Complete compartmentation of these three management functions is difficult in definition and is virtually impossible in practice. Certainly the control process is dependent upon the skill and thoroughness of the organizational and planning efforts. However, it is the control aspect that promotes success and permits the realization of success by measurement and reporting for sound direction of operations.

Among the most effective board implementation in this area are program plans, financial budgets, formal reviews of actual performance as opposed to planned performance, and careful appraisal of differences between the two. Departures from plan and budget must not go unexplained and unjustified.

Inadequate control over resources soon dissipates or prevents financial efficiency. The resource control aspect of management includes the improvement of efficiency through error reduction, quality maximization, and reduction of costs. It also should protect resources through deterrents to waste, defalcation, and loss of assets.

Board Operations

Boards that operate with full regard for and are effective in organizing, planning, and controlling should find the process of motivating staff and board members to be immensely facilitated, if not entirely accomplished. However, board actions in meetings and members' actions outside of meetings are motivational to staff and board either positively or negatively. Board actions or operations may be divided into three general areas: trustees' orientation and education, conduct of meetings, and other communications.

Orientation and Education

Management audits of Texas MHMR community centers have revealed board education as one of the major weaknesses in the past. Board education continues to be a problem in many present centers, in that actual practice does not yet follow approved policy, however excellent.

The content of trustee orientation and continuing education efforts is beyond the scope of this paper, but three related provisions are needed in regard to new appointments:

1. Trustees should be informed in advance as to training expectations.

2. Trustees should be appointed sufficiently in advance for certain orientation *prior* to the effective date of appointment. (Many trustees think that at least three months and three or more board meetings are needed for the average person to become an effective trustee.)

3. Orientation in program content, facility tours, and acquaintance with key staff should never be optional, as is the case in a few centers.

Boards coordinating with their appointing authorities to obtain these requirements may have difficulty maintaining the maximum membership of nine, but could function more effectively with fewer, better informed, more committed trustees.

Board Meetings

Severe time limitations, the many complex issues faced, and the varying viewpoints presented by individuals and organizations in the community require competent management of board meetings and advance utilization of standing committees and staff assistance. Typically, community center boards in Texas have three or four standing committees responsible for these functional areas: programs, personnel, planning, budget and finance. Community relations may require another committee. Ad hoc committees may be appointed as needed.

The obvious need for structured agendas (advance issuance of relevant papers, adherence to parliamentary procedures, and maintenance of official minutes for all meetings) is generally accepted for committees as well as for board meetings. Orientation for new board members should include a review of the above matters, and an opportunity for any members inexperienced in committee meetings or board-governance procedures to enhance their knowledge. Even then, inefficient, ineffective board meetings may result because of personal or group dysfunction. Some of the causes have been enumerated as:[4]

1. Frustrations with the agenda, insufficient information, and feelings of powerlessness.

2. Group conflict, personal feelings regarding the leader(s), and unspoken determination to block agenda items or group purposes.

3. Lack of communication skills, poor listening, shyness, and aggressiveness.

4. Polarization, apathy, fear of decision-making, and poor leadership among other issues.

A few boards have had occasional difficulty in obtaining a quorum. Certain boards have addressed this problem in positive fashion: their bylaws require the resignations of trustees not attaining attendance requirements. Why not similarly treat other trustee inadequacies that regularly impair board or center effectiveness?

Board/Staff Communications

Boards have been found to need a definition of acceptable trustee communication policy, both with staff and with persons outside the centers. Good leadership often "sees a center through" in this regard, but turnover and training needs warrant explicit coverage of the subject in board bylaws or other policy statements. Examples of abuses that can otherwise occur are:

1. Individual trustees sometimes "speak for the board" without its prior knowledge or authorization.

2. Staff may ask for advice or even a decision from an individual trustee without board concensus or the executive director's knowledge.

3. An individual trustee not officially authorized may seek information privately of staff.

4. Social or other board/staff contacts may result in the unauthorized, unreported exchange of information and/or views.

Any of the above can obviously conflict with the best interests of a center, its staff, and the trustees.

In the Texas centers that are well regarded operationally, boards administer and control as a body only, and primarily with written, officially approved policies and directives, including the minutes of its meetings. Quoting from one center's board policy manual, "The authority of the Board results from the group action . . . No individual . . . member has any authority . . . (Guidance) of the organization (center) can only be . . . by the full Board acting in an official capacity." It is important for staff morale and management effectiveness that board policy in this area be clearly stated. Such policy should not prevent needed communication between key staff members and the board or any of its committees. Staff, with the chief executive's knowledge and concurrence, should be available for consultation to any authorized board representative. However, it is important that *directives* from the board not be formulated or communicated in these contacts. Figure 2 is a graphic presentation of the relationships, oversimplified, considered most appropriate between board and staff in board meetings.

In regard to written communications, it is axiomatic that the larger an organization, the more formality is needed. Any public organization, subject to the constant scrutiny of its constituents and funding agencies, should give special attention to publishings and other records. Staff members and trustees sometimes have had negative experiences in establishing or following published organizational policies. There definitely is an art in defining and writing effective policy statements, but the principles involved have been aptly stated:[5]

1. The statement of any policy should be definite, positive, clear, and understandable to everyone in the organization.

2. Policies should be translatable into practices, terms, and peculiarities of every organizational unit.

3. Policies, regardless of how fundamental, should not be inflexible; they should, however, possess a high degree of permanency.

4. Stability of policies is essential.

5. Only as many policies as necessary to cover anticipated conditions should be in effect; too many become confusing or meaningless.

6. Policies should be predicated on fact and sound judgment, not personal reflections.

7. Policies should rarely prescribe detailed procedure.

8. Policies should be compatible with the public interest, recognize economic principles, and conform with the laws.

Conclusion

Boards should concern themselves primarily with top-level concerns of service delivery in the community, and should use available

Regular Board Meetings

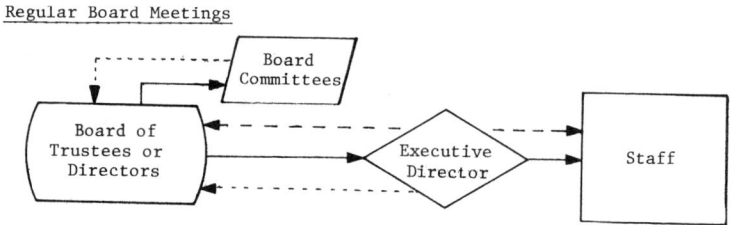

Quarterly Reviews + Workshops

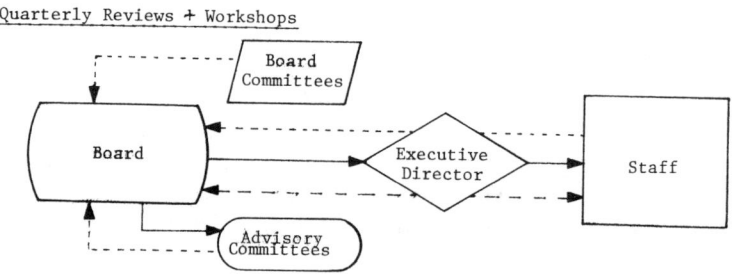

Planning & Budgeting Meetings

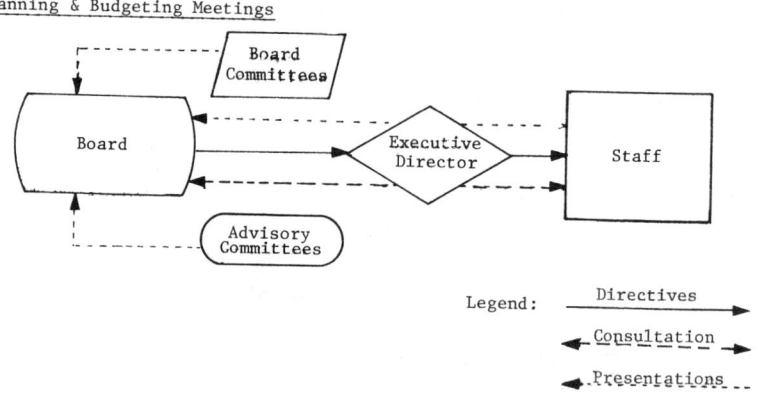

Figure 2
Board/Staff Communication

resources as responsibly and efficiently as feasible. Accomplishment of this goal in the public sector requires concern, knowledge, skill, and organization at the board level. Ideally, the board will not deal with the day-to-day administration of the center. Trustees who insist upon doing so can better serve as volunteer assistants to the center staff.

Adequate organizational efforts, sound planning, and proper control measures require competent board members, capable board leadership, and key staff assistance. The results are predictable: a competent staff, good morale due to strong motivation, and center effectiveness in delivering the services to community residents in need. The latter is the fundamental and only important reason for the existence of a center.

References

1. *Resource Manual for Boards of Trustees of Community Mental Health and Mental Retardation Centers in Texas.* TDMHMR and the Hogg Foundation Mental Health, 1977, pp. i, 8–1.

2. Hersey and Blanchard. *Factors in Managing Behavior in Organizations.* Prentice-Hall, 1969.

3. Robert N. Anthony. *Planning & Control Systems.* School of Business Administration, Harvard University, 1965.

4. Leland P. Bradford. *Making Meetings Work.* University Associates, 1976, pp. 20–33.

5. Paul E. Holden. *Production Handbook.* The Ronald Press Company, 1948, p. 1383.

The Aftermath of a Hurricane: What One Mental Health Center Did Following a Major Disaster

William H. Simpson, Ph.D.

Hurricane Frederic, with winds of 145 miles per hour, struck Mobile, Alabama, the evening of September 12, 1979. The winds continued until 3:00 A.M., as people crouched in shelters while their world whirled around them: power was out, water was disrupted, roofs and bridges disappeared, and trees blew like matchsticks with ever-present crashing sounds.

Mobile was dark and under seige. The only communication that night came from one radio station managing to function with emergency equipment. As morning came this once bustling city was quiet, stunned and immobilized by the destruction that was far more widespread and severe than predicted. People came from their homes, walked around in a stunned silence, and went back inside. Only later in the day did they emerge for the clean-up chores at hand.

More than 33,000 families suffered significant loss of housing, property, or income. Miraculously, only four people died as a direct result of the hurricane. The destruction was estimated at $2.5 billion, the largest in history. Typically, hurricane severity is measured by the number of deaths inflicted, so Hurricane Frederic by this standard could not be termed a major hurricane. The residents of Mobile, Alabama, however, think otherwise.

Physical destruction can be assessed and repaired, but more important are the human damages, which are much more difficult to measure, evaluate, or repair.

The Mobile Mental Health Center was active throughout the storm, during the cleanup period, and the following recovery. The morning after the hurricane nothing moved, for streets were impassable, so the Center staff was not able to assemble until the second day following the storm. About a dozen of us reported for work on that day, principally the management staff, and began an assessment of the situation from the standpoint of Center services and its role in the aftermath of the disaster. The pharmacist in the drug program somehow managed to arrive by bicycle on the morning following the storm, and he issued the methadone dosages to those drug clients who reported to the program. A number of the clients were waiting on the steps of the drug center, anxiously awaiting their prescribed dosages.

On the second day after the hurricane, we made contact with the Civil Defense Office and subsequently were assigned to the Welfare Department according to the State "Disaster Plan." However, our role was defined as one of issuing food stamps and filling out forms for receiving relief. This activity did not appear to be an appropriate utilization of experienced mental health professionals, so we subsequently were assigned to the Disaster Relief Centers working under the auspices of the American Red Cross. Our crisis team members were immediately dispatched to the emergency shelters. The management staff met daily to assess the previous day's work and to determine proper courses of action for the next day. These daily debriefing sessions aided in charting a course of action until such time as we were able to establish a formal disaster counseling program through the National Institute of Mental Health and the Federal Emergency Management Agency. Our own clients slowly began to emerge from the refuge and to request service. However, these requests did not get heard until the week following the hurricane. For the most part, these early contacts were those patients involved in the medication clinic or follow-up program.

By the end of the second week, most of our staff had been accounted for, and while many had suffered severe damage to their homes and personal property, all managed to maintain some degree of normalcy in their work schedule and home repair schedule.

At this point in the hurricane aftermath (the end of the second week) the Center was maintaining two operations: its general program and its special services in the disaster emergency shelters.

Frustrations with obtaining the necessities of life brought on many crises in the immediate aftermath. Water and electricity were unavailable, as was telephone service. Most streets were completely impassable, and gasoline was a not-to-be-found item. These frustrations brought on encounters. One crisis team member found herself an arbiter of a confrontation between a law enforcement officer and a relief worker. She sent the officer home to sleep and the worker to a quiet room. In the days following, counseling was as much evident to relief agency staff as to clients and general populace.

The governor established a curfew to deter looting. This 7:00 P.M. to 7:00 A.M. time frame helped manage the situation. Looting came under control quickly through enforcement of the National Guard.

The American Red Cross reported the following destruction as a direct result of Hurricane Frederic: 690 houses completely destroyed; 31,060 houses with major structural and exterior damage; 23,304 houses with minor damage; 3,907 mobile homes destroyed; 1,703 with major damage; 35 apartment units completely destroyed; 46 apartment units with major damage; 773 apartment units with minor damage; 31 small businesses were destroyed; 10 disaster-related deaths; and 3,315 disaster-related injuries and illnesses.

As the Center worked with local agencies and its clients, maintained its regular programs, and carried on activities at the shelters, a call was received from the Alabama Department of Mental Health, asking if we were in need of any assistance. Our initial response was to report that we did not, since we were able to account for all personnel, assess damage to the facility, and keep our programs underway. However, the Department of Mental Health was not to be denied, and a team of people (composed of office staff and representatives from other mental health centers in the State who volunteered to help) traveled to Mobile to assess the situation and the operational status of the Center. As all motels and hotels were either damaged or occupied by insurance adjusters from across the nation, as well as construction crews, the Site Team members were housed in the residential section of the Drug Abuse Treatment Center. They remained several days, moving around the community and making their assessment of the situation. They concluded that the entire staff "looked like hell," and that we engaged in a considerable amount of suppression, concerning our own feelings following the hurricane. In the Site Team's debriefing they recommended that we file for a Disaster Grant with the National Institute of Mental Health and allowed us an opportunity to view ourselves through their eyes. We concluded they were correct.

An initial survey of Center clients immediately following the hurricane revealed some trauma as a result of the storm, but a preoccupation with obtaining life's necessities and a desire to reestablish their lifestyle overwhelmed other concerns. The most common reaction was one of fear and anxiety. Within the weeks and months immediately following the storm, the trend seemed to move more toward depression and anxiety. Within those few days and weeks afterwards, people were considerably less tolerant and tempers were unusually short. One interesting symptom that was widely observed was the obvious increase in automobile traffic. The entire population appeared to need to stay mobile. Streets remained clogged from early morning to late evening. This delay could be partially attributed to debris still existing on most streets, but even taking this into consideration, there appeared to be the need to remain mobile, even with gasoline prices 10 percent higher.

Following the visit by representatives from the Alabama Department of Mental Health, the Center received consultation help from the National Institute of Mental Health and was advised of directions needed to secure a Disaster Counseling Grant. Subsequently, such a grant request was submitted and later successfully awarded for a period of six months. The extent of the damage resulted in the slow processing of the grant, so the award did not come until approximately five months after the disaster. The Center did encounter some criticism for the late receipt of such a grant, but the delay was a bureaucratic one, i.e., processing the application through the various levels of government and departments, Alabama Department of Mental Health, National Institute of Mental Health, and Federal Emergency Management Agency. The Center thought everything was proceeding on schedule, so you can imagine our surprise when a call was received from a representative in the *local FEMA Office*, requesting further documentation of the need for the grant!

The Disaster Counseling Grant enabled the Center to establish three outreach teams to provide screening diagnosis, needs inventory, counseling, follow-up, referral, and consultation. Following the receipt of the grant, we advertised the eighteen positions and received 225 applications. This response serves as a reflection of the then current economic situation of the area. Fortunately, this large number of applications allowed us to select eighteen individuals, whom we divided into three teams. A team was placed in each of the three "high destructive areas" of the county. The initial step, following selection of the staff, was the location, rental of office space, and equipment acquisition. We had to integrate the project with our main information data system and so certain input forms had to be developed. The next stage involved a training program for the staff. This training was secured through the University of South Alabama Continuing Education Center. In our opinion, this training was essential to what became a successful implementation of the project; particularly in view of the fact that the staff performing the duties were, for the most part, paraprofessionals. Even though we were being pushed to implement services, we felt the training program was essential to the skill and understanding necessary for the community consultant counselors and to the schedule of the grant.

Each team was composed of three individuals, a team leader, and two consultant counselors, and secretarial support. The teams reported to a Project Director. The Assistant Area Supervisor and Team Leaders were employed at a master's degree level and the Counselor Consultants were bachelor level individuals. The initial meetings on community awareness of the project brought many people who wished the Center to become advocates for the disaster victims. While in the beginning our expectation was that advocacy was to be a small activity, it turned out to be a large part of the work of the counselor consultants.

Our approach was not to publicize the program through the media, as we felt this would generate a great many referrals and contacts, and we would simply not be able to provide the services requested. This rejection would give this project a negative impact, rather than a positive one, and with that in mind, we formed an Advisory Committee composed of representatives from community agencies. We worked with them in the implementation of the program. During the early weeks of counseling, contacts were mainly from Civil Defense, Red Cross, Small Business Administration, and the Department of Pensions and Security. Cooperation from these agencies enabled the team to advocate some definite, tangible assistance to community residents, as well as some individuals who were having difficulty helping themselves. The Advisory Committee provided important guidance and timely advice about service delivery during the project. At monthly meetings, the Advisory Committee kept the staff informed of policy changes and community resources, suggesting effective and appropriate policies for service delivery.

At the time of this writing, the project has received over 800 individual referrals, and has made over 2,900 contacts with clients. In addition, the counseling teams have made over 1,800 contacts with agencies and community organizations on behalf of the referrals. The counselors have helped hurricane victims deal with stress (due to storm-related unemployment),delays in processing recovery assistance applications, contract fraud, and delays in home repairs; helped locate temporary housing; and counseled families with problems. The counselors have been supportive and informative and, when necessary, have advocated positively and productively for the referrals. Most of the clients were women who were young, adult, married, and had low income. Half were from minority groups, and the major presenting problem was economic in nature.

Counseling teams have been involved with groups of hurricane victims adjusting to new living conditions. The teams have recently organized groups of adults and children to deal collectively with recovery problems, to share common experiences following the disaster, and to facilitate group solutions to common problems. A major problem for residents in temporary, crowded housing trailer parks resulted in developing alternative living plans and group needs. Coordinated and facilitated by various team counselors, these process meetings were effective media for these families in exploring possible resources.

Referrals to the counseling teams have been equally divided among self-referrals who learned of the service through word of mouth (33%), agency or community organizations' staff referrals (32%), and others such as friends, physicians, clergymen (35%). Generally, the initial contact is a phone call or office visit, which is followed by an appointment with the counselor to determine what service is needed and can be offered to the client. There are usually two contacts prior to accepting a referral officially. It is during the initial contact that information is gained as to whether or not the problem is hurricane related. Analysis of about 500 cases result in the following breakdown of services provided at the time of initial contact: screening diagnosis (22%); information/referral (32%); crisis counseling (14%); client advocacy (19%); other, including information gathered, (13%). Analysis of the 800 cases provides the following breakdown of presenting problems: agitation/depression (6%); acting-out behavior (1%); confusion/disorientation (1%); request for advice (52%); request for medical aid (2%); other, i.e., request for advocacy, recovery assistance, etc., (36%).

The teams' response to client's needs vary from short-term counseling to extensive advocacy work on the part of the families unable to help themselves create alternatives for recovery. By August 1980 there were many families who still had not taken steps toward recovering from the hurricane. Over 100 families were awaiting individual or family grant awards; another 100 had recently received their awards, but the repairs to housing had not yet begun. A six-month period of wet weather in the area since the storm increased damage to many homes, so that the original estimate of cost was insufficient. Moreoever, hundreds of families still remained in temporary housing, and the number of calls received from these trailer parks to the counseling center increased daily. At this point those victims who had not achieved stability got worse, not better.

It should be noted that the Team responded to the victims' plight not only on the telephone and at the office, but at the victims' homes and in other places such as field locations or community agency headquarters.

During the time that the disaster counseling service was continuing, the Center's comprehensive services program was restored to full operational condition. We did experience some growth in cases during this time, with hurricane-related emotional problems. In addition, during early spring, our community experienced two floodings that included much of the same area affected by Hurricane Frederic. The plight of the people became further compounded, particularly those for whom repair and reconstruction had not yet taken place. Almost a year later, we were finding families and areas where no assistance was given and the plight of the people was little changed from the day after the hurricane.

There are recommendations and plans that were derived from our experiences following the hurricane. Among these are the following:

(1) A community mental health center (CMHC) should have a disaster recovery plan on record, which is updated periodically in conjunction with other community agencies. While the disaster recovery planning may fall to another agency in the community, the CMHC should take an active role in the development of the plan.

(2) The disaster recovery authority does not accurately perceive the role of the CMHC in the recovery program. Actions are generally taken to assign CMHC staff to inappropriate roles. The appropriate roles for such trained staff should be defined in the plan.

(3) During the period immediately following a major disaster, the center's patients will divert their attention to restoring their lifestyle and creature comforts. The demands for service will typically be those related to the grief and depression following the disaster, particularly if there has been a large number of deaths.

Part II
Psychiatric Outpatient Treatment
in the 1980s

Foreword to Part II

John T. Salvendy, M.D.

Following a rich tradition, this section contains the written version of papers presented at the Eighteenth Annual International Meeting of POCA, which took place June 5–7, 1980, in Toronto, Ontario. It also includes an essay by John Furedi, M.D., Ph.D., whose guest paper was designated for a later POCA meeting but included here for informative purposes.

The theme of the conference "Psychiatric Outpatient Treatment in the 1980s" indicates the main area of thrust. However, a number of contributors broadened the scope and added meaningful insights into the psychological, sociopolitical, scientific, and legal aspects of outpatient psychiatry.

Due to unfortunate circumstances beyond the editors' control, the essays by F. Lowy ("Psychotherapy in the 1980s") and J. Flannery and G. Taylor ("Integrating Mind and Body in the 1980s") could not be included in this volume.

The articles in this portion are not designated to offer comprehensive coverage of all treatment modalities but rather selected reviews, analyses, and forecasts in a number of important areas in psychiatric ambulatory care. Prominent American and Canadian authorities reflect the contemporary "state of the art" in their treatises. Common to most papers is a balanced presentation of theory and applicability to clinical practice.

Azima achieves this integration in her lucid focus on child and adolescent services.

A quasi-historical survey by Brown (delivering the Opening Address) of political dynamics in the Far East during the Second World War has an astonishing relevance to our understanding of contemporary international affairs.

Freeman presents the art of the possible in the delivery of commu-

117

nity-based services and yet manages to come up with truly innovative recommendations.

Furedi describes the evolution of psychiatric outpatient facilities in Hungary—an interesting contrast to the North American scene. An in-depth analysis of the present situation and the future trends in the drug management of the largest chronic ambulatory population—the schizophrenics—is presented by Lapierre.

The POCA Award recipient for 1980, Professor Heinz Lehmann, M.D., is one of the great pioneers in the field of psychopharmacology. His seminal work has allowed in the first place the enormous expansion of extramural care to a vast segment of the psychiatrically ill. His keynote address about the story of psychopharmacology is as fascinating in its clarity as the man himself.

Renshaw gives us a concise summary of the theory and practice of sex therapy. Her open and lively style is designed to encourage mental health professionals to learn more about this increasingly important modality.

Salvendy discusses a gamut of controversial issues in group therapy with the intention of shedding light on some important misconceptions.

Mental health legislation as it affects the management of the psychiatric patient is scrutinized critically by Swadron who was instrumental in drawing up the innovative Mental Health Act 1967 in Ontario.

Last but not least, the late Jack Weinberg delivers an elegant and challenging tour de force on the dynamics of aging. If anyone ever could integrate the psychosocial, cultural, and biological aspects involved and win more than a lip service for the elderly, Weinberg has done it!

Planning and practice in mental health disciplines has been characterized for the past several years and is likely to be for the foreseeable future in terms of limited resources and emphasis on treatment and rehabilitation. The contributions in this section reflect this realistic orientation without losing faith in the viability of less than grandiose solutions.

Multi-author compilations have been often criticized for uneven quality. The editors hope that the readers of this section will find all the carefully chosen topics informative and stimulating.

Acknowledgements

I would like to express my appreciation to Dr. Bertram S. Brown, at the time of the Conference Assistant Surgeon General, United States Public Health Service, for his acceptance to deliver the Opening Address on a short notice and to Mr. John Graves, Director of the Clinical Meetings Department of Wyeth Limited, for his valuable technical advice and assistance. For all the work involved in preparation of these manuscripts I wish to thank my secretary, Mrs. Anne Eberle.

Last but not least I am grateful for the constant support of my wife Elfi and my children Sylvia, Daniel, and Oscar who individually and collectively kept my editorial morale high!

JOHN T. SALVENDY, M.D.

Psychiatry in the 1980s

Bertram S. Brown, M.D.

It was a pleasure to participate in the annual meeting of POCA in Canada, a country that has a very special meaning for me. My father, who had first emigrated to the United States from Russia at the age of seventeen, in midlife and at about the same age I am now, after raising his family in New York City, emigrated to Canada. At that time I was out of college and my sister still in high school. He spent twenty-five years in Montreal (my sister graduated from McGill) until his retirement. He had become a Canadian citizen, so for my whole adult life I have been living a sort of Canadian-U.S. identity, I might even say identity crisis.

It is very difficult to fit into somebody else's shoes, as when you take an exam and the smart students still answer what they know best rather than what the professor asks. It has to appear to be what the professor asks, but it is still best to write about what you know. This essay examines psychiatry in the 1980s in an international perspective.

Since I left the directorship of the National Institute of Mental Health a little over two years ago, I have been spending most of my time at the Woodrow Wilson International Center at the Smithsonian Institution. The first year was spent as a scholar studying the U.S.-U.S.S.R. health and science exchange, particularly in psychiatry, since for five or six years I had been the chief United States psychiatrist working with Andrei Snezhnevsky in the schizophrenia exchange, part of the overall exchange in heart disease, cancer, the environment, and the like. In that setting there was the chance to dig deep into understanding the nature of the similarities and differences in the practice of psychiatry in the United States and in the Soviet Union. Jack Weinberg, past president of the American Psychiatric Association, was the heroic and international figure at the 1977 Honolulu meeting when the Declaration of Hawaii was passed, which condemns certain abuses of psychiatry. For the past year, after finishing the scholar phase, I have been Director of Symposia and Seminars and have gone more broadly into international spheres. Can we take on the task of predicting the future? If we're going to predict the future, we're going to have to start to think about the future. How does one do that? As you know, in terms of futures, there are new journals, clubs, cults, religions, and people who are serious futurologists. As either practitioner or administrator, organized, disciplined dealing with the future is a critical but neglected component. I have been working with an organization that is of significance to POCA, the National Association of Private Psychiatric Hospitals, studying the structure of their boards of trustees—what the boards are like, what they do, etc. It was evident that the critical deficiency was in long-range planning. Similarly, the American Psychiatric Association has recently established a long-range planning committee (for the late 1980s and the 1990s) and is devoting real resources to the task.

Long-range is defined as "more than five years," which is in such stark contrast to the corporations and the military, where long-range planning is serious and intense and helps to illuminate the immediate crisis of the day as well as next year's budget. The "scenario" technique is used very often. We must realize that in planning scenarios or thinking about possible scenarios, we will be confronting what is called the non-Euclidean law. The non-Euclidean law says that all straight lines, when projected, sooner or later curve up or down or wiggle, which makes it a little difficult. Then there are the new lines that come out of nowhere and yet regularly appear on the map. Those are the two laws of long-range planning.

I would like to discuss, in the perspective of an international overview, some of those projected lines that might appear on the graph as we look at psychiatry in the 1980s and beyond. If you are going to look at the future, you do have to decide whether it is five years or ten or twenty. Each year there's another good excuse for projecting the future. In the United States, 1976 was a period when by symmetry or the law of parity a 200-year projection was made. In 1975, the predictions were for the quarter of a century remaining.

My first big-league attempt to project the future was back in 1966, when the Group for the Advancement of Psychiatry (GAP) had its twentieth anniversary. You may remember that GAP was formed on the floor of the APA in 1946, where the "old fogeys" were thrown out by the young "revolutionaries." The young revolutionaries had become middle-aged and were going through a midlife crisis. I was too young to understand their crisis, but they decided to do something really astonishing and invite a young person to talk to them about the future. Thus I was asked to give that twentieth anniversary speech. It was published a couple of years later as "Psychiatric Practice and Public Policy."[1] If you will pardon speakers who like to quote their own words, let's hear what they sound like fifteen years later.

What can psychiatry do now, what should it do soon, what must it do in the future? While it is blatantly grandiose to presume that psychiatry will make the poor, rich; the bad, good; the intoxicated, sober; the unhappy, happy; it *is* fair to ask what we can contribute to these compelling human hopes. For while the demands are insatiable, and the crescendo call cannot be met in its totality, we *must* look in turn at each of these areas and see what we can or cannot do. We must not pull our heads back into the turtle shell of the medical model.

It is not only the delineated area of mental illness that concerns us, nor even the amorphous matter of mental health, but an evanescent and evolutionary concept that encompasses both illness and health—the quality of life. This shift in focus was clearly expressed by Dr. Alan Gregg on the 100th anniversary of the American Psychiatric Association in 1944, when he predicted "You will be concerned with the optimum performance of human beings as civilized creatures."[2]

As we deal with these matters, the special position of psychiatry becomes clear, for we are marginal men who live between our roots in the mechanisms of biology and our branches in the flowering of the intellect and emotion. We are trained to hear the thump of the human heart through a stethoscope in our ears. We move on to listen to the collective cry of mass malfunction and misery; from the strident scream of the urban riot to the distant wail from the migrant labor camp, and above all to the millions and billions who are hungry.

When I read the above I do not know whether to blush or be proud, for the call was certainly for a bold and expansive social psychiatry and a fearless, if not grandiose, proposal to deal with the psychiatric aspects of hunger and famine. My first prediction, then, from my international and global perspective, is that the psychiatric aspects of famine and hunger will be a major theme of the mid- and late 1980s. I know of only one psychiatrist who is devoting major professional attention to this issue—Dr. David Ratnavale, a Sri Lankan, who is now at NIMH as a visiting scientist. He has been studying the psychiatric and mental health dimensions of malnutrition, hunger, and starvation as well as problems facing refugees (in the United States and camps overseas) and personnel involved in their relief, rehabilitation, and resettlement.

The year was an important year for me, since that was when I was appointed Director of the National Institute of Mental Health. At issue there was not being a seer, not looking into the future, but actually trying to mold the future. One criterion for judging whether or not that future was indeed molded was my attempt at leadership by announcing three key priorities in my first forty-eight hours: (1) the mental health concerns of children and youth, (2) the mental aspects of law and order, and (3) mental health concerns for minority groups. I will not go into (1) and (3). Much happened. Not enough for the mental health of children and youth, but much happened. And much happened in the area of mental health concern for minorities. But I think it is more instructive to focus on the failure—the mental health concerns of law and order, the relationship of psychiatry to crime. When I announced that priority, my closest colleagues and friends said "You're a fool. It can't be. You don't know what you're dealing with." Remember, there was a president named Nixon and an attorney general named Mitchell. Nevertheless, I formed a task force of Law Enforcement Assistance Administration and NIMH professionals. I remember a 1971 key meeting in Denver, where we were going over the relationships of a law enforcement organization with a mental health organization. It was the time of the Manson murder trials and Air Force One was delayed in the air for an hour before landing in Washington because President Nixon had just announced, before the trial, that Manson was guilty. It took 45 minutes for his staff to wiggle out of that one. What a dramatic anticipation of the future that was!

I did not really understand the problem of what I would have to work with, and many attempts were made without much success. As I look back, I think the reason for the failure was that I had identified and worked with the wrong group: the criminals and the perpetrators. I had not identified that the victim and the victims would be the real organizational groups that would make a difference in mental health concerns. And that is what happened. Starting in the late 1970s victims began to organize themselves. Rape victims were the first and a National Center for the Control of Rape was created. The elderly people who were being victimized began to organize themselves and started the movement for the Concerns of Older Americans. Right now the field of victims is emerging as a new major area for mental health. A recent edition of the journal *Evaluation and Change* is totally devoted to victims.[3] The titles of the articles in this particular issue (Appendix A) highlight a major change, and in this sense it will have practical impact in terms of your own programming for the 1980s.

At this juncture let's take an imaginative leap and do something crazy, almost psychotic, with the time machine. We've gone back to 1966 and 1970, talked of 1980, focused on 1990. I'd like to pretend that 1980 now, was 1970 then, and I am in my thirties. I have just become Director of the National Institute of Mental Health and I have to choose priorities for molding major mental health and psychiatric services for the 1980s. What should I do? The answer is crisp and clear. I would choose the psychiatric aspects of the handicapped and disabled. I choose this example because I do indeed predict that there will be a major significant social movement that will shape psychiatric care in the 1980s. Over the past several years, in the United States and in many other countries, the organization of handicapped individuals has become a social movement. For instance, the United States focus is leading to marked changes in the laws and regulations. It is such a strong movement that counter articles are appearing to fight it. The demands of handicapped and disabled persons for access and the arguments you read about in the press have to do with wheelchairs and ramps and physical barriers and buses, but the barrier on the physical level is nothing compared to the barriers on the psychological and psychiatric levels. How many clinics have services for the deaf? Or the blind, or the cerebral-palsied, or the paraplegic, or any of the other 220 organized handicapped groups? It is for this reason that I predict that since this *ought* to be, whether molded by the handicapped or by others, it *will* be a major movement in the 1980s.

The United Nations has declared 1981 as the International Year of the Disabled Person. There are councils now forming in Canada and the United States to carry out related activities. In the United States a group of us are doing a subproject on psychiatric aspects of handicap and disability, and we are looking across the world for others working in this area. We would very much like to hear from anyone doing work in specific handicaps and their psychological and psychiatric aspects.

We've gone now from different aspects of predictions, to time machines, to a touch of international perspective. Let us go into the issue of international perspective with a little more discipline and thought and put psychiatry itself—the field, including of course some of the allied professions as part of that field—under scrutiny.

Psychiatry is a growing subspecialty of the field of medicine. Across the world it varies in size from nearly 10 percent of the medical profession in the United States to less than one tenth of one percent in many parts of the developing world. The United States has one psychiatrist for every 10,000 people; India has one psychiatrist for every one million people. Psychiatry is a profession dealing with both clear and overt mental illness, as well as with the distress and behavioral disturbances of the problems of living. The balance of effort and activity within this vast spectrum varies from country to country and from culture to culture. Insofar as psychiatry deals with, or takes a role in, the "problems of living" arena, there are not and never can be enough psychiatrists. There are about one hundred thousand psychiatrists in the world, over half in the United States and the Soviet Union. If this were a measure, the world would have half a million psychiatrists. The debate as to what is the proper balance in dealing with these two arenas, clear illness and the problems of living, is the most universal debate in psychiatry in both the developing and developed world. This debate has dimensions that relate to the internal self-identity and searchings of the profession, a debate that stems from the impact of societal demands. It is only poorly understood. When psychiatry has taken on dealing with life's miseries, it is indeed a new church replacing religion, as well as a replacement for other social structures that served these purposes in the past.

At the 1976 Vancouver meeting of the World Federation for Mental Health, two of the great minds in the field debated: Ivan Illich, author of *Medical Nemesis,*[4] and Morris Carstairs, a leading psychiatrist. They discoursed about churchman versus doctor, pastor versus psychiatrist, and at one point Illich said, "We have medicalized life. We were born to suffer." And Carstairs said, "The doctor's first job is to relieve suffering." There was no end to that debate.[5] It just clarified the issues for all of us.

The role of psychiatry in the realm of sociopolitical leadership has become equally controversial and unresolved. Some psychiatrists clearly feel the profession has a major role in such arenas as prevention of war, dealing with poverty, race, sex, hunger, while others feel efforts in these broad issues overstep both the capabilities and boundaries of psychiatry. In medicine, and particularly in medical schools, psychiatry has become the defender and keeper of the humanistic traditions. Psychiatry's foundations are psychology and biology (the latter now referred to as the "neurosciences"). Some of the social sciences, particularly sociology, have become part of the framework. However, two major areas, cultural anthropology and sociology, are only recently being considered as either making a contribution to or influencing the field of psychiatry. Of special note is that culture affects biology as clearly as it impacts individual personality and social systems. This influence takes place through nutritional patterns and mating patterns affecting genetic pools or perhaps even affecting fundamental operations of the brain.

We know that both country and culture are critical in defining normality and in shaping symptoms and patterns of illness. Frequent syndromes include susto, latah, imu, koro (all related to fear), amok and other rages, and a variety of changes of states of consciousness, yielding a variety of possessions and trances, such as kitsunitsuki. Carrying the concept of culture to include political and social systems, we can see that culture clearly shapes the health and mental health care delivery systems. Following are a few examples.

I was asked to consult with Japan by its government. I have been in Japan many times, and it is a long story to describe how one gets to be asked to Japan to consult with the government. They had a fascinating, spiralling crisis. Japan has about 100 million people, the United States has 200 million, so it is easy to think of a graph in terms of one to two, roughly 2 to 1. After World War II, Japan had less than 100 thousand psychiatric beds, about 80 thousand. No one knows exactly how, but after World War II it started to climb, climb, climb and is now 370 thousand beds. During that same period the United States went from 600 thousand psychiatric beds to 200 thousand. Can you picture that curve—80 thousand to 370 thousand, 600 to 200? Japan has four times as many beds per capita as the United States and the numbers are still climbing. What's behind the phenomenon of so many psychiatric beds in *the* country? (Japan is now number one in per capita income and in 1979 produced more cars than the United States, 9 million.) Two major dimensions emerge from this analogy, one is straight finance; the government has a wonderful insurance program, which really covers the doctor's bills. There are no state systems, so any psychiatrist worth his salt opens a mental hospital as an entrepreneur. Eighty-three percent of the psychiatric beds are private, fully funded, and that's why my colleagues, at least in the United States, are sometimes puzzled that I don't have total enthusiasm for national health insurance. I've seen what lack of controls can do.

The second dimension is cultural. It is still "shameful" in Japan, more so maybe than in the United States and Canada, to be mentally ill and hidden away in a hospital. Outpatient care is not yet quite accepted, and this interplay of the cultural and the financial aspects begins to explain some of the phenomena that take place and can cause large changes in such patterns as outpatient and inpatient care.

Let us switch to another example where an international perspective begins to give clarity to thoughts of what will happen in the 1980s and 1990s. Focusing on Soviet psychiatry, the question to ask clearly is, "What does one learn from looking at psychiatry in the Soviet Union in the broad context of Soviet studies?" One of the best-known books on this subject is *Psychiatric Terror* by Bloch and Reddaway,[6] a document about the use of psychiatry in the Soviets' handling of dissidents. The very phrase seems an overstated propagandist's polemic. However, in the context of Russian and Soviet history studies, one finds terror a common continuing fact. Terror has been used in the titles of a number of eras and epics: the terrors of the pogroms before the revolution, the Stalinist terrors, and other periods called just that. Terror becomes an instrument of state. From that perspective, terror loses its polemical quality and becomes a phrase in a more sober and frightening context, making the issue worthy of careful study. This point brings us to the issue that is most important to all of us, the relationship of psychiatry to the government, to the state. One begins to think about the role of the government, to see glimmers of understanding of the law's relationship to psychiatry. One begins to get glimmers of what anti-psychiatry and the patients' rights movement are about. As I have studied psychiatry and looked upon it as a science, I have realized more and more the importance of the utilization of science in achieving the purposes of the state. This relationship between the sciences and the state is more familiar in atomic engineering, space efforts, and military science. A recent book by the exiled Soviet dissident Zhores Medvedev is called *Soviet Science* and covers the issue in great detail.[7] His writings, and others I have studied, provide powerful statements that illuminate, in my opinion, when psychiatry will be misused. *I declare that when a state, meaning its government, feels its vital interests are at stake, it will use its full powers—and convert means if they prove necessary—to retain its office and achieve its goals, including the misuse of psychiatry.*

There are examples in the United States which I am free to quote. The psychiatric hospitalization of General Walker during our civil rights riots, is one example. There are several others: the rifling of Daniel Ellsberg's psychiatrist's files is a good example of the lengths to which the state will go, such as misusing the mental health professions when it feels its security or well-being is endangered or threatened. There is a longer, more dramatic example of the misuse of psychiatry by a government. In 1973 I made an extensive tour of Japan with my then Executive Assistant, K. Patrick Okura, a prominent Nisei, and with philanthropist Philip Hallen. It was a full month's visit and provided me with a grasp of Japanese affairs which I had not had before. Since then I have made several visits. The high point of another visit in 1978 (concerning the Japanese psychiatric bed crisis) was a meeting and discussion with Dr. Takemi, president of the Japanese Medical Association (which is comparable to being the president of the AMA) and the Assistant Secretary for Health, a combined post he had held for 27 years. If you think of that society and the guru and the sword and the samurai and the boss, that's the sort of position he had. We were Dr. Takemi's guests over a lengthy luncheon, along with a small group of elders who determine in great measure who will be the Minister of Health, the real governing power. We discussed many of the health and policy issues concerning the United States and Japan. And we discussed such things as physicians' incomes and fees, the role of pharmaceuticals and drugs, a whole host of subjects. He then asked about my current endeavors, and I told him I was studying the U.S.-U.S.S.R. health and science exchange. The time of my visit coincided with the impending signing of the Japanese-Chinese friendship treaty. The Soviet Union did not want Japan to sign the treaty, which had been in negotiation for five years, and there was great sensitivity around the relationship of Japan and the Soviet Union.

In the above setting I described some of my interests and concerns about U.S.-U.S.S.R. psychiatrists, psychiatry, and their relationships to one another. The question of the misuse of psychiatry entered the conversation, and then Dr. Takemi looked toward me and said, "This is what we did in World War II to those who disobeyed the Emperor." This fascinating and tantalizing statement led me to several days of exploration. That was a part of World War II that had so far been undescribed.

I am oversimplifying, but from 1938 to 1941, before Pearl Harbor, Japan had a War Party and a Peace Party. The War Party was led by General Tojo, the only man ever to be Japan's Chief of Staff and Prime Minister at the same time (1941–1944). The War Party overcame the Peace Party in 1941, as history so obviously shows, and the decision to attack the United States was made. This result leaves the question of what happened to the Peace Party and the generals who were its leaders. The Party disappeared and it was not widely known that many of the generals spent World War II in psychiatric hospitals as places of incarceration.

During my discussion with Dr. Takemi these facts were not known in the United States. When I returned in August I was able to talk with many historians who are now working to get the documentation and descriptions of this particular use of psychiatry at a time of crisis in a national culture. Of particular interest is that one of the Peace Party generals who spent the war in a psychiatric hospital testified at the War Crimes trial following the Japanese surrender. There was a smaller war crimes trial like the trial at Nuremberg. The general testified against General Tojo and was present when Tojo was executed.

I give the above as an example of some of the ways we must think about psychiatry in the 1980s. You are going to have the feeling that there are lines coming out of the chart which you do not expect. New major uses of the government and the courts, new groups of people and organizations (such as victims), new aspects of the organization of population groups, new problems around immigration and migration. The clearest way to think about it is that psychiatry and psychiatric care will be affected profoundly by such events and by any political-social-economic developments. And as these events unfold, let us be prepared to adapt to them and, whenever possible, to mold them to our basic value system, to our basic beliefs, and to our basic religion (which for me is to care for the sick as well as to prevent mental illness when we can) and to promote the quality of life for all.

References

1. Brown, B. S. Private practice and public policy. *American Journal of Psychology* (August 1968), 125(2): 489–495.

2. Gregg, A. A critique of psychiatry. *American Journal of Psychiatry* (1944), 101, 285–291.

3. Salasin, S., & Davis, H., eds. *Evaluation and Change,* Special Issue, 1980. Minneapolis Medical Research Foundation and National Institute of Mental Health.

4. Illich, I. *Medical Nemesis.* New York: Pantheon Books, 1976.

5. Beiser, M., Krell, R., et al., eds. *Today's Priorities in Mental Health: Knowing and Doing.* Academic Debate: Menninger, C., Illich, I., & Carstairs, G. M. Be it resolved: There is no need for mental health professionals, 229–259. Miami: Symposia Specialists, 1978.

6. Bloch, S., & Reddaway, P. *Psychiatric Terror; How Soviet Psychiatry Is Used to Suppress Dissent.* New York: Basic Books, 1977.

7. Medvedev, Z. *Soviet Science.* New York: W. W. Norton, 1978.

Outpatient Therapeutic Servicing of Children and Adolescents: Review and Preview

Fern J. Cramer Azima, Ph.D.

Review

In the last two decades there has been a marked impetus to treat emotionally disturbed children and adolescents on an outpatient basis and to deinstitutionalize the treatment program and setting. Originally, the concept of intervention, assessment, and therapy followed the model of the traditional child guidance clinic, where the designated child was assigned to one therapist, and the needy parent to another staff person. This model in the large majority of instances has given way to the clinic-team where the family is seen as a unit and assessment and treatment procedures are shared and planned from in-take to discharge.

The impact of group and family therapies, and the increasing competence of the paraprofessional team on the one side and the increasing sophistication of the consumer, altered significantly the procedures and feedback to the family, to the school, and to the community. It also became clear that a certain proportion of significantly disturbed children needed more than once-a-week therapy, and emphasis was put on treatment in day hospitals or therapy day centers. This fact was compounded with the increasing costs of hospitalization. There was also the parallel rationale that the child and adolescent would normalize and be reintegrated more quickly if not separated from his family or peers. Presently, hospitalization is used where the illness is very grave, medication under supervision is needed, and separation from the family is indicated.

Currently, the emotionally disturbed child and adolescent may be seen individually, with family, in a group, or with peers and geographically may be treated in a hospital, outpatient clinic attached to a hospital or based in a community home, or the school. This order is correlated with the degree of pathology and normality (Hersov & Bentovim, 1977).

It became clear that many seriously disturbed children previously hospitalized could be treated in a day center (Connell, 1961; Rafferty, 1961; Dingman, 1964; Chazin, 1969; Gritzka, 1970; Bentovim & Boston, 1973; Ross & Schreiber, 1975; Bauman, 1976).

A treatment sharing of psychotherapy, recreation, music, arts and crafts, exercise, and education was among the needs seen to match the deficits in the child's development. In addition to the psychiatrist, psychologists, and social worker, educators, special care counselors, occupational therapists, and often other paraprofessionals joined the staff of these clinics (Vaughan, 1963).

For these intensive day hospitals to function adequately most authors referred to the need for an intact or at least cooperative family (La Viètes et al., 1965; Marvin, 1967). In some instances, intensive day treatment was seen as a partial enforced separation from the family, for example, a model half-way between once-a-week therapy and that of complete hospitalization; this treatment provided links to and from inpatient treatment and follow-up for the child and his/her family (Marshall & Stewart, 1969). It is to be noted that in this review facilities for autistic or psychotic children (Fenichel et al., 1960) have been minimally included and deal primarily with the child who exhibits reactive, behavioral, and developmental disorders. It would seem, however, that more disturbed children including the borderline are being serviced by outpatient facilities. Increasingly, schools began to identify the high-risk child (Anthony, 1970, 1974; Weintraub et al., 1975). The dilemma was how to withdraw the child from the academic milieu and yet prevent lags in cognitive development. Two procedures were evolved, namely to incorporate the school into the clinic or to bring the psychotherapeutic facilities into the school (Godwin et al., 1966; Graffagnio et al., 1970; Blom, 1972; Weintraub et al., 1975; Whittaker, 1975; Victor & Halverson, 1976).

Outpatient services were increasingly demanded by the community to treat the less seriously disturbed or "maladjusted" youth (Schonfield, 1971; Grégoire & Normandeau, 1980) or to provide information relating to birth control or drugs. With the increasing expertise of educators and paraprofessionals, schools and recreational programs became broadened by combining psychodynamic and/or behavior therapy principles. The latter focused on well-identified symptoms and briefer interventions (Ross, 1974; Leventhal & Weinberger, 1975; Lillesand, 1977). During the 1960s and early 1970s there was a rush of "drop-in-centers" for addicted youth. It soon became clear that some of those adolescents were too seriously disturbed to be treated in the community and were referred to psychiatric in- or outpatient facilities.

Therapeutic Servicing

A limited survey of the literature of outpatient services for the age group of three to eighteen reveals that the child or adolescent is screened alone or with his/her family and that the treatment plan is more and more planned by the total team. Many modalities and admixtures are used including individual, family, peer duos (Bender, 1976), group therapy with use of projective modalities (Azima, 1959; Abramowitz, 1976), television (Martin & Parrish, 1973), puppets and drama, mutual storytelling and squiggle (Stephenson, 1973).

Several authors have addressed themselves to the differences in treatment modality for the latency child (Sarnoff, 1976; Anthony, 1976) as compared to the adolescent (Rafferty, 1961; Blos, 1979). Elsewhere I have outlined that therapies of children involve a combination of nonverbal play and activity with gradual transition to works and symbolization. Therapies with adolescents differ significantly from both those of children and adults, specifically their ambivalence and attack on authority figures, and other resistances that evoke strong countertransference reactions in the therapist (Azima, 1971, 1976, 1977).

Research

The marked difficulty in conducting research in psychotherapy outcome is well known, and in studies with children these problems are compounded by such factors as testing the less articulate child, the biased inaccurate reports and recall by ambivalent parents, fewer available instruments for assessing change in this age group, and the clear difficulty in teasing out which changes are due to the programs and which ones to the child's own development during this time period (Levitt, 1971; Robins & O'Neal, 1971; Robins, 1972; Anthony, 1975). Heinicke and Strassman (1975) commented on the dearth of adequate research and suggested some effective ways to evaluate outcome. Hersov and Bentovim (1977) reviewed inpatient and day hospitals and concluded that there were good results with young children who shared manifest anxiety, fear, and separation problems, while there were poorer results with those who showed character disorders, psychotic disorders, or severe speech and language problems. Differences in outcome favoring early intervention have been documented by Chess and Thomas (1972), and Gersten et al., (1976) has dealt with the issue of stability and change in children and adolescents with behavioral disturbance.

Heinicke and Strassman (1975) in a careful clinical study pointed to the fact that longitudinal follow-up revealed positive outcomes not seen at the point of discharge or first assessment. Gold and Reisman (1970) revealed a two-thirds (2/3) improvement rate in a community-based treatment unit school but found that the children often needed continued school and therapy follow-up. Leventhal and Weinberger (1975) reported in a four-year follow-up that a brief therapy program was highly effective. Baumann (1976) reported that in a thirty-one month follow-up of sixty-two children, fifty-two were in public school. A case-by-case comparison of the fifty-two children revealed significant "intrapsychic growth development" for thirty-two of the children. Abramowitz (1976) reviewed the overall effectiveness of group therapy with children.

We (Azima & Laroche, 1980) have evaluated a four-year intensive Therapy Day Center (TDC) for emotionally disturbed latency-aged children of the Royal Victoria Hospital. This facility is a multi-tiered intensive psychoeducational day program servicing a small group of twenty children; the program may be conceptualized as a "developmental integrative link" in the treatment phase (Azima, 1977). Parents are a mandatory part of the treatment program, as well as school and community consultations. The treatment team consists of a child psychiatrist, two psychologists, a social worker, a special care counselor, and three teachers. Additional personnel are provided by undergraduate or graduate students from the various disciplines who are engaged in field placements.

Originally, our intention was to offer a brief intensive day therapy experience of approximately six months to children whose primary problems were emotional and reactive and who fell within the normal range of intelligence. In general, our referrals have been from schools for impulse-ridden boys and girls, who act out, are disobedient, and cannot learn under the usual classroom situation. The sad, isolated child is not routinely referred until bizarre behavior at school or at home is readily apparent. More frequently we are seeing the borderline child who has managed to a certain degree to function until a debilitating stress occurs. Deprived and abused children are now more easily recognized by the educator and are quickly referred.

In general, the children seen at our center have a low self-esteem and act out defiantly. Learning disabled children are seen only if this problem is secondary to the emotional ones. Our short-term therapy goals have proved difficult to achieve so far, and our programs now extend for at least two years intensively, and then with less frequent follow-up. Our experience has demonstrated that at times the pathology of these children is so extensive even by the age of seven that it cannot be modified by a brief intervention. The TDC program has evolved through various strategies experimenting with a clinic classroom for two years and subsequently with two classes in a neighborhood school.

Presently we have (1) an intensive half-day program four times a week for children six to eight. This group receives a variety of psychotherapies and teaching within the clinic setting. (2) A partial integration program—for those children who are able to function in the school setting, either in a special class or later in a regular class, and who attend the clinic one or two half-days a week in groups for social skills, socialization, and psychotherapy. (3) For older children functioning in their home schools, a half-day psychotherapy program is provided. (4) Consultation to schools prior to acceptance, active liaison during the program, and follow-up following discharge are provided by the professional team. (5) A parent program is mandatory and involves them in groups, individual sessions, and child-parent therapies. Because of the numerous single parents, they are at times considered a separate group. Approximately every two months the parents meet with the codirectors and treatment team to review and give feedback on their own child's progress. At these meetings we attempt to integrate our information from the parents, school, and community.

The goal of the day center for the child or teenager is to provide a structured program with a high ratio of staff per child, which allows pleasurable and confident socialization with peers and gradual progression of enrichment, competence, and mastery in the areas of play, sport, recreation, and school activities. Psychotherapy with individuals, in groups, and with families is interwoven according to specific needs of the child. Within the overall scheduling, the curriculum is individualized to allow the specific problems of the patient to be addressed by each staff member. There needs to be a very frequent feedback, coordination, and planning system with all team members to maximize the therapeutic milieu for the children. Where possible, the group composition allows the maximizing of identification and normalization in the presence of some ego strong children by the modeling of the competent, consistent, and sympathetic staff.

When rivalries and splittings develop among team members and are not quickly and well resolved, the child continues to respond as in the dysfunctional family. Whittaker (1975) has spoken cogently of the "ecology" or focus of the child treatment as more important than the locus, be it residential or day treatment; he states that the basic purpose of both settings is to foster a family support system rather than the isolation of the child and to involve the parents as equal partners in the helping process.

The specifics of the helping process must be concretely detailed and "demystified." There is general agreement that there must be parallel change within the parents to allow a new acceptance and integration of the disturbed child within the family system. Involvement in this program has made us increasingly aware of the pros and cons of integrating the emotionally disturbed child into the regular classroom. Some highly disturbed children should not attend school until a certain level of stability can be demonstrated. Integration back into the mainstream must be done slowly and carefully. The addition of a month's summer camp has proved a very valuable therapeutic experience for this population. Teachers, special care counselors, and students plan field trips, swimming, sport programs, etc., to encourage learning and sharing with the group of peers in a less structured, more true-to-life setting. There are new insights of the children during this camp period, and at times they have made unexpected gains.

Another helpful aid to our program has been the use of the one-way screen and television. Both groups are curious about, stimulated by and impressed with the TV playback of their performances, which frequently they wish to change or correct. Again, the group viewing the film heightens the pressure for attention and analysis of behavior. The teaching and supervisory aspects of the videotapes are most helpful. Throughout the program, various children are given special attention outside the clinic by a "buddy" who most frequently is a McGill University student who has volunteered his or her time.

It is the experience in this day center and with the program with adolescents that provides the background for the formation of my predictions for outpatient servicing for the age group five to eighteen in the 1980s.

Preview

My discussion here is aimed at giving some suggestions to fill some voids in the present outpatient servicing for youth and to meditate on the problems that will face us in the 1980s in the treatment of children affected by the changing culture over the last twenty years.

Expansion of Psycho-Educational Clinics

There is a continuing need for innovative models within the educational system to accommodate the emotionally disturbed child. This change will necessitate increasing expertise for educator and psychotherapist to find ways within and outside the normal classroom to motivate and stimulate the child's mind. Some children function best in a permissive, free setting, highlighting arts, music, and dance while others are better in structured, competitive, strict ones. It is not only the match of the setting but also, and more realistically, the expertise and competence of the teachers and mental health consultants who cooperatively seek solutions to such problems as boredom, carelessness, dropouts, rage, and destruction of school property and physical violence when disciplined. Striking, dissatisfied teachers simply collude with the resentful angry child. Within some school systems there is often a split between guidance personnel and the educator, whom they interpret as judgmental. Similarly, the invading consultation team often is seen as threatening and castigating. The territories of what is the school, home, and community and where and what interventions should be made are still being defined. Such rifts must be healed to guarantee success in this area.

Our present theories of general system consultation, liaison, and follow-up interventions have helped significantly to open the boundaries between school and outpatient clinics. The fusion of cognitive theories, social-psychological theories of parent-child rearing, and psychodynamics would seem to be a fertile field for this decade of newer approaches to conceptualizing innovative treatment modalities.

More specifically, some children cannot be maintained in the school setting and should be treated and taught in the outpatient clinic until such time as a return is possible. Alternative time streams within the school program, independent of the formalized year or grade requirements, would make for easier exit and reentry.

Another high priority is the early identification of the high risk child. Intensive mental health mobile clinics coordinated with school personnel should routinely visit preschool, kindergarten, and the first grade at least once or perhaps twice a year to help in this early detection phase. Rapprochement between the disciplines helps each to define the overlapping roles of cognition, psychodynamics, and the earliest recognition and referral of the disturbed child.

Integrated Networks of Outpatient Treatment Facilities

It is likely that there will be a more holistic approach to the continually disturbed child, adolescent, and the family.

In our work it has become apparent that there is a network of services that are often not integrated—such as the school, court, police, community and social service, or foster or group homes. Integrating such services necessitates an administrative member of the outpatient team. We have designated this function to the team leader, the member who assumes the primary therapist role. This member becomes the "keeper of the file" and the liaison with the parents, school, and staff. This vigilance for the child shapes the philosophy of sharing and caring and downgrades professional team rivalries.

To make our programs more effective there needs to be an agreement at the point of intake where the child and his/her family will be best serviced. Because of the increased sectorization approach (the division of the city into specific subdivisions from which the treatment center draws its population), this communication is at times difficult. The repercussions of deinstitutionalization even in the youth area happened because corresponding community resources or rehabilitation areas have not been provided. The projected network would consist of identification of the needy child at Station A in the community or school. The decision then is whether to assess the feasibility of treating the child at this level or to refer the child to Station B—to a learning disability clinic, to placement in a foster or group home, or to a psychiatric outpatient clinic. Upon discharge the child and the family are referred to Station C—a rehabilitation or halfway center within the community. If a crisis reemerges the child can be quickly rerouted. Brochures would then be prepared about the existence of these treatment areas and central contact points for the parents.

At this juncture it may be relevant to discuss the lack of good, small group homes for the latency-aged child who cannot function either at home or in regular foster homes. Finkel and Thomas (1971) and Rubinstein et al. (1978) have addressed this point, and the latter present an interesting parent-therapist program in which five healthy nuclear families have treated 115 children with a mean age of nine and a half years since 1972 for an average stay of 18.7 months. They found it facilitating and cost effective. However, within the confines of a therapy day center that is limited to space and staff and where the children are significantly disturbed, it is at times difficult to decide whether the presence of the children's parents or volunteer "normal" untrained parents would be a help or a hindrance. The possibility of separating a child from the family even for a brief three-week residential group home placement has been extremely therapeutic at times, if planned and carried out in close liaison with that facility and the parents.

The centralization of the child and family charts possesses the dilemma of confidentiality and intrusion into the individual's privacy in an increasingly socialized state. In many areas parents are entitled to read the charts and at times may be unprepared for their contents. The resulting trend might be the watering down of the facts into superficialities.

The holistic approach, tried in a few places (and not the subject of this review), may expand and contract for all of the medical, psychological, social, and legal issues of the patient and the family at the point of first contact.

Preventive Referrals

Rarely is a child referred to a mental health facility until a problem of some severity has developed, and yet in retrospect it is clear that there are many life crises through which the child and the family would have been helped and perhaps a traumatic scar prevented or diminished. Here one thinks of referrals from lawyers who witness pathological family wars, divorce, financial gains or losses, death and division of property, and guardianship; from the clergy who witness a host of trauma too numerous to list; from our own hospital personnel who must explain parental loss, severe illness, impending surgery, and handicap to the child; from the police and from the schools who become suspicious of neglect and abuse. In this latter area physical abuse and rape have been so widely discussed that they are quickly reported more and more by neighbors, family members, and at times by the child himself. Yet psychological abuse, which shares most of the same insidious dimensions, is still just whispered about or kept behind locked doors. Within our clinics we are aware of seeing only the tip of the iceberg; if one child in a family is a risk, the other siblings are likely to be also.

Changing laws now allow adolescents to be treated, in some areas, without parental consent. New social legislation will be forthcoming in the 1980s to protect the rights of the child.

An area of considerable risk continues to be the family and child who immigrate from a culture, dystonic from our own. At times immigration officers and religious leaders are the first to hear the stories of families who cannot cope and wish to return home or who have no recourse but to fall emotionally ill.

Many readers may decry that I may be suggesting that the floodgates of referral will be opened too wide. These suggestions, however, are born of seeing children who unfortunately have waited too long. What I am suggesting here is an outpatient therapeutic modality that offers liaison service on a brief transitional consultation basis.

Research

The difficulties in carrying out psychotherapy research in the area of childhood has been touched upon earlier in this paper. Yet there is a high priority for the development of new assessment instruments including interaction measures; outcome and longitudinal studies of day treatment programs; comparison studies of the offspring of manic-depressives, schizophrenia, and delinquent parents; comparison of the efficacy of different psychotherapy and behavior therapy approaches for defined age periods from early childhood to late adolescence; predictive studies on high risk children, etc. We must progress from the global epidemiological studies of the vulnerable child (Shepherd et al., 1966; Graham, 1978) to the careful assessment of the quality of mental health care and the degree to which changes seen in the treatment program generalize outside the clinic, how long they remain stable, and under what circumstances old or new conflicts arise.

One-way screen and video equipment are helpful in clinical procedures and provide invaluable communication data as well as training procedures that may be reviewed for changes before and after varying therapeutic interventions. These films are in great demand in beginning programs here and abroad. Portapack TV is used in our program in both clinic and school settings to study intensively the children's and teachers' interaction, changes in aggressive behavior, etc. Another collection procedure is the use of cassettes or tapes on which the children record in the clinic, the school, and specifically the home their dreams as they awake, their concealed thoughts and feelings, which often they cannot reveal to the therapist.

Fortune-Telling for the 1980s

How are our children and adolescents prepared for this decade? They are the children of parents who rebelled against the atomic age and overthrew the Victorian superego and dread of the future. The final blow for the great establishment was seen in their gluttonous use of drugs, their long hair and faded jeans, rock and roll, and Woodstock. They dropped out of school, lived in communes, and returned to nature as happy flower children. Educational standards became increasingly permissive—exams were graded pass/fail, and children were taught to be astute gamblers on multiple choice questions. The grandparents looked the other way and admitted that they had not run their world very well. Crushing blows for obedience to authority figures were served by disillusioned soldiers, the assassination of a president and a presidential candidate, and the eviction of another who had cheated in the highest post of government. Television programs pumped the images of sex symbols, bionic men and women, fantasies of exploring space with robots to carry out every whim. Parents and educators who were part of the anti-order era were now faced with their own disobedient grandiose children.

Many times these children were made to accept parental roles, to run the one-parent family, to become the housekeeper, to arrange the evening meal of take-out pizza served in front of the wide screen, and to mix a drink or prepare a joint for the father or mother upon their return at night. Suddenly they were asked at the stroke of eight to become good children, to do their homework, and to go to bed and have nice dreams.

To this condensed psychohistorical college one may add the new search for religion and cult leaders to replace parents and provide happiness, success, and protection. Against this backdrop one may perhaps wonder if the syndromes of narcissism and borderline pathology have not been encouraged by these multiple stresses and the breaking of traditional family bonds. There was a search for instantaneous cure.

The pendulum partly began to swing back in the late seventies. The concepts of marriage, family, and children gained renewed interest. Women who had remained barren until age thirty-five rushed to have children. Society began to reassert its traditional values. The seventies ended with a celebration for the Year of the Child and a pledge to look after him/her much better for the years to come. Yet it may indeed be bewildering for the most normal child to face some of the leftover turmoils listed above. Although many promises have been made, the backlash against the pampered child and the bravado adolescent may even be more severe for this decade.

Conclusion

An overview of the literature places the outpatient servicing of children in historical perspective with reference to the major designs, locus of the clinics, types of therapeutic servicing, and some relevant research investigations. The Therapy Day Center of the Royal Victoria Hospital is described briefly to illustrate the details of how an actual outpatient children's service functions. The preview section deals with anticipated growth in the expansion of the psycho-educational clinics, in integration of the networks of outpatient treatment facilities, in preventive referrals, and in future research. A final section is devoted to some future fortune-telling for the eighties, for inevitably the impact of cultural crises affect the expression and style of the emotional disorders in any time period.

In concluding this review and preview it is clear that the type of latency child seen in the fifties has changed considerably. In our clinics we will likely be facing even more precocious youths on the one hand and on the other, children who are bored, depressed, or unmotivated. Referrals to children and adolescent outpatient services will not decrease in the eighties. The stresses may become different but it is hoped that we will be better equipped to solve some of the problems by heeding some of the messages of the past and by integrating clinic teams with frequent feedback to parents, school, and community. A high priority is necessarily placed on outcome research studies to specify thrust of our clinical servicing to emotionally disturbed children and adolescents.

References

Abramowitz, Christine V. The effectiveness of group psychotherapy with children. *Archives of General Psychiatry* 33:320–326, 1976.

Anthony, E. J. The treatment of the latency child. *Canadian Psychiatric Association Journal* 21:199–209, 1976.

Anthony, E. J. (ed) *Explorations in Child Psychiatry; The Use of the Series Experiment in Child Psychiatric Research*, pp. 381–416. New York: Plenum Press, 1975.

Anthony E. J., & Koupernik, C. *The Child in His Family; Children at Psychiatric Risk* (Vol. 1). New York: John Wiley & Sons, 1970.

Anthony, E. J., & Koupernik, C. *The Child in His Family; Children at Psychiatric Risk* (Vol. 3). New York: John Wiley & Sons, 1974.

Azima, Fern J. Transference-countertransference issues in adolescent group psychotherapy. In N. S. Brandes & M. Gardner (eds.), *Adolescent Group Psychotherapy*. Science House, 1971.

Azima, Fern J. Group therapy for latency children. *Canadian Psychiatric Association Journal* 21:210–212, 1977.

Azima, Fern J. Therapeutic interventions and countertransference in adolescent and latency age groups. Proceedings of International Forum of Psychoanalysis, Berlin, 1977.

Azima, Fern J., & Laroche, Catherine. Evaluation of a therapeutic day centre for emotionally disturbed children. 1980.

Azima, H., & Cramer-Azima, Fern J. Projective group therapy. *International Journal of Group Psychotherapy* 9:176–183, 1959.

Baumann, Evelyn. A day treatment program for severely disturbed young children. *Hospital and Community Psychiatry* 27:174–179, 1976.

Bender, Barbara. Duo therapy; a method of casework treatment of children. *Child Welfare* 55:95–108, 1976.

Bentovim, A., & Boston, M. A day centre for disturbed young children and their parents. *Journal of Child Psychotherapy* 3:46–60, 1973.

Blom, G. E., Ekanger, C. A., & Parsons, P. C. A psychoeducational approach to day care treatment. *Journal of the American Academy of Child Psychiatry* 11, 13:492–510, 1972.

Blos, P. *The Adolescent Passage; Developmental Issues*. New York: International Universities Press, 1979.

Chazin, R. M. Day treatment of emotionally disturbed children. *Child Welfare* 48:212–218, 1969.

Chess, S., & Thomas, A. Differences in outcome with early intervention in children with behaviour disorders. In M. Roff, L. Robins, & M. Pollack (eds.), *Life History Research in Psychopathology* (Vol. 2). Minneapolis: University of Minnesota Press, 1972.

Connell, P. H. The day hospital approach in child psychiatry. *Journal of Mental Science* 107:969–977, 1961.

Dingman, P. R. Day hospitals for children. In R. L. Epps & L. D. Hanes (eds.), *Day Care of Psychiatric Patients*. Springfield, Ill.: C. C. Thomas, 1964.

Fenichel, C., Freedman, A. M., & Klapper, Z. A day school for schizophrenic children. *American Journal of Orthopsychiatry* 30:130–143, 1960.

Finkel, N., & Thomas, S. Group homes for school age children in day care. *American Journal of Orthopsychiatry* 42:252–253, 1971.

Gersten, J. C., Langner, T. S., Eisenberg, J. S., Simcha-Fagan, O., & McCarthy, E. D. Stability and changes in types of behavioural disturbance of children and adolescents. *Journal of Abnormal Child Psychiatry* 4:111–127, 1976.

Godwin, M. P., Conner, M. E., Atkins, S., & Muldoon, J. F. The role of the educational program in psychotherapeutic day care centres for children and teenagers. *American Journal of Orthopsychiatry* 36:345–346, 1966.

Gold, J., & Reisman, J. An outcome study of a day treatment unit school in a community mental health centre. *American Journal of Orthopsychiatry* 40:286–287, 1970.

Graffagnino, P. N., Buckman, F., Orgun, I., & Leve, R. Psychotherapy for latency age children in an inner city therapeutic school. *American Journal of Psychiatry* 127 (5):626–634, 1970.

Graham, P. J. Epidemiologic perspectives on maladaption in children; neurologic, familial and social factors. *Journal of American Academy of Child Psychiatry* 17:197–208, 1970.

Gratton, L., & Pope, L. Group diagnosis and therapy for young school children. *Hospital and Community Psychiatry* 28:188–190, 1972.

Gregoire, J. C., & Normandeau, S. A community approach for youth with adjustment problems. *Canada's Mental Health* 27:4–7, 1980.

Gritzka, K. An inter-disciplinary approach in day treatment of emotionally disturbed children. *Child Welfare* 49:468–472, 1970.

Heinicke, C. M., & Strassmann, L. H. Toward more effective research in child psychotherapy. In M. Rutter & L. Hersov (eds.), *Journal of the American Academy of Child Psychiatry—Modern Approaches*. Toronto: J. B. Lippincott Company, 1977.

La Vietes, R., Cohen, R., Reens, R., & Ronall, R. Day treatment centre and school; seven years experience. *American Journal of Orthopsychiatry* 35:160–169, 1965.

Leventhal, T., & Weinberger, G. Evaluation of a large scale brief therapy program for children. *American Journal of Orthopsychiatry* 45:119–133, 1975.

Levitt, E. Research on psychotherapy with children. In A Bergen (ed.), *Handbook of Psychotherapy and Behavior Change*, pp. 474–494. New York: John Wiley & Sons, 1971.

Lillesand, Diane. A behavioural psychodynamic approach to day treatment for emotionally disturbed children. *Child Welfare* 9:613–619, 1977.

Marshall, K., & Stewart, M. J. Day treatment as a complementary adjunct to residential treatment. *Child Welfare* 48:40–44, 1969.

Martin, C., & Parrish, M. The application of closed circuit television instant replay as a self-confrontation method in children's group therapy. *Corrective and Social Psychiatry and Journal of Applied Behavior Therapy* 119 (2):31–35, 1973.

Marvin, B. The significance of the parental force in psychotherapy with disturbed children in an open residential setting. *Child Welfare* 46 (a): 514–521, 1967.

Rafferty, F. T. Day treatment structure for adolescents. In J. H. Masserman (ed.), *Current Psychiatric Therapies*. New York: Grune & Stratton, 1961.

Robins, L. N. Follow-up studies of behavior disorders in children. In H. C. Quay & S. Werry (eds.), *Psychopathological Disorders of Childhood*. New York: John Wiley & Sons, 1972.

Robins, L. N., & O'Neal, P. The strategy of follow-up studies with specific reference to children. In J. G. Howells (ed.), *Modern Perspectives*. New York: International Child Psychiatry, Brunner/Mazel, 1971.

Ross, A. L. Combining behavior modification and Groupwork techniques in a day treatment centre. *Child Welfare* 7:435–444, 1974.

Ross, A. L., & Schreiber, L. S. Bellfaire's day treatment program; an interdisciplinary approach to the emotionally disturbed child. *Child Welfare* 3:183–194, 1975.

Rubenstein, J., Armentrout, J., Levin, S., & Herald, D. The parent-therapist program; alternative care for emotionally disturbed children. *American Journal of Orthopsychiatry* 48:654–662, 1978.

Sarnoff, C. *Latency.* New York: Jason Aronson, 1976.

Shephard, M., Oppenheim, A. N., & Mitchell, S. Childhood behavior disorders and the child-guidance clinic; an epidemiological study. *Journal of Child Psychology and Psychiatry* 7:39–52, 1966.

Schonfeld, W. A. Comprehensive community programs for the investigation and treatment of adolescents. In J. S. Howells (ed.), *Modern Perspectives in Adolescent Psychiatry,* pp. 483–504. New York: Brunner/Mazel, 1971.

Stephenson, Susan. Working with 9 to 12 year-old children. *Child Welfare* 6:375–382, 1973.

Vaughan, W., & Davis, F. Day hospital programming in a psychiatric hospital for children. *American Journal of Orthopsychiatry* 3:542–544, 1963.

Victor, J. S., & Halverson, C. F., Jr. Behavior problems in elementary school children; a follow-up study. *Journal of Abnormal Child Psychology* 4:17–29, 1976.

Weintraub, S., Neale, J. M., & Liebert, P. E. Teacher ratings of children vulnerable to psychopathology. *American Journal of Orthopsychiatry* 45:838–845, 1975.

Whittaker, J. K. The ecology of child treatment; a developmental educational approach to the therapeutic milieu. *Journal of Autism and Childhood Schizophrenia* 5:223–237, 1975.

The Story of Psychopharmacology— Past, Present, and Future

Heinz E. Lehmann, M.D.

In the year 1955 an unexpected and dramatic phenomenon surprised and delighted officials at the Mental Health Office in the state of New York. The rate of annual increases in the resident population of mental hospitals (a rate that had been constantly rising every year until it had reached an all-time high in 1950) suddenly reversed its course and started dropping. Previously, there had been no indication of any slackening of pace of its rise, and at that time mental hospital cases had doubled since 1929, over-crowding had reached 33 percent, and the existing shortage of 23,000 beds seemed bound to increase by 2,000 or more each year.

Yet, in 1955 to 1956 this ominous, apparently inescapable upward trend was halted and from then on, for quite a few years, changed into a fall of mental hospital populations (Brill & Patton, 1959).

Two other phenomena were observed at the same time: first, the mental hospital inpatient population began a downward trend in 1955, not only in the state of New York but on the whole North American continent. Second, the rate of patients treated in psychiatric outpatient clinics rose explosively and, between 1960 and 1968, almost quadrupled in the United States (Berger, 1972). As a consequence, the role of outpatient treatment for psychiatric illness, a role that was insignificant only 25 years ago in comparison to that of mental hospitals, today far surpasses in importance that of the hospitals and the private sector.

Coincidental with these events there was the sudden development of a new and powerful therapeutic weapon in psychiatry. Psychotherapeutic drugs had been used for the treatment of mentally and emotionally disturbed people throughout recorded history, but the

148

effects of these drugs had been unreliable and had lacked any scientific rationale. More important, there had never been any drugs that could eliminate the symptoms of true madness, such as hallucinations, delusions, or mental incoherence, and could help those patients who had lost all contact with reality.

Such drugs were discovered and their clinical usefulness demonstrated in the years between 1950 and 1955, and there is little doubt that this was the essential factor, even if not the only one, that turned the tide toward the fall in mental hospital patients and the consequent extraordinary rise in importance of psychiatric outpatient treatment a quarter of a century ago.

It is for that reason that I chose to review the story of psychopharmacotherapy and psychopharmacology. A detailed and comprehensive account of the history of psychopharmacology would take much time and would become rather technical and dry; therefore, I shall try to present a brief overview of what has happened in this field and what the physicians' and scientists' abiding interests and successful achievements were at various periods of time.

Psychopharmacotherapy and Psychopharmacology

Psychopharmacotherapy is a clinical discipline, based mainly on empirical observations, while psychopharmacology is a scientific discipline that is founded on systematic research, critically evaluated evidence, rational theory, and logical conclusions. For most of the time of the development of these two disciplines, the achievements of the clinical branch of psychopharmaceutics, i.e., psychopharmacotherapy, ran ahead of those of scientific psychopharmacology. However, as we shall see later, during the last fifteen years or so, academic psychopharmacology with a sudden, brilliant outburst of new discoveries, sophisticated theories, and complex instrumentation seems to have outstripped the success of clinical psychopharmacotherapy.

Psychopharmacotherapy: Historical Review

In Figure 1 I have tried to represent the different successive achievements of modern psychopharmacotherapeutics for the last 140 years. The time course is recorded on the horizontal axis while the ordinate is divided into measures from one to ten, according to arbitrarily chosen values of the historical importance of the various discoveries. I chose 1840 as the beginning, because it was during that time that the first major breakthrough occurred in psychopharmacotherapy with the discovery of general anesthesia. Using nitrous oxide, ether, and chloroform, doctors then, for the first time, conquered *pain* completely, at least for certain periods of time, as Morton proved in the Massachusetts General Hospital in 1848, when he successfully performed the first ether anesthesia during a major surgical operation. General anesthesia then became a new medical technology that in turn enabled surgery to make its own rapid progress. Further milestones in the fight against pain were the discovery of local anesthesia with cocaine by Köller and Sigmund Freud in 1894, and the introduction of the all-purpose analgesic, acetylsalicylic acid (aspirin) by Dreser in 1899.

Freud, as is well known, also was aware of the pleasantly stimulating effects of cocaine on the central nervous system. He used the drug to obtain those effects frequently himself and wrote to his fiancée how he could hardly have stood the boredom at certain evening parties that he attended had it not been for the beneficial action of cocaine. However, it soon became clear to him that cocaine was neither an innocuous stimulant nor, as he had believed at first, a cure for patients who were addicted to morphine, but had addicting and dangerous properties of its own. He quickly abandoned its use and from then on mistrusted and disliked psychoactive drugs all his life, although he also predicted in his writings that many of the psychological symptoms that at his time could only be treated with psychoanalysis would be treated someday with chemical substances (Freud, 1964).

The first phase of psychopharmacotherapy that had concentrated on the conquest of pain, was soon followed by another that was characterized by an attack on insomnia. In 1857, Locock introduced the bromides into therapy. They were originally used as anticonvulsants but later became the first medical tranquilizers and for many

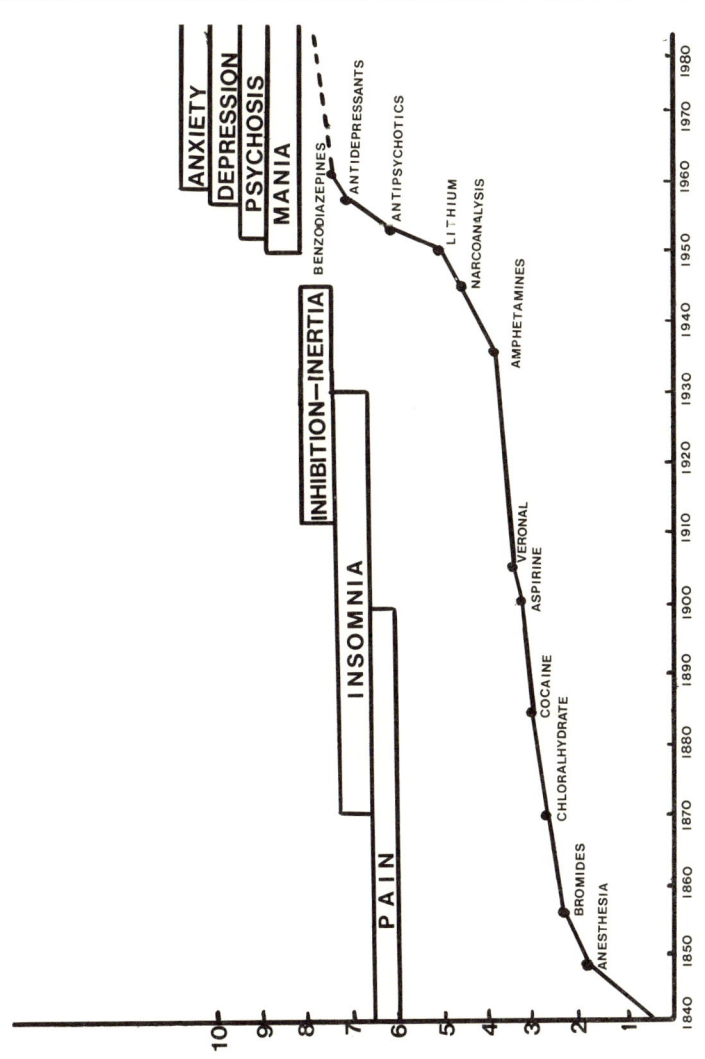

Figure 1
Psychotherapeutic Drugs
Historical developments of psychotherapeutic drugs and their
relative importance from 1840 to the present

years were prescribed as treatment for anxiety and insomnia. However, they were not very effective and also highly toxic, so they are hardly ever prescribed any more. Interestingly, their anticonvulsant action, which is real, was suspected by Locock because potassium bromide was known to reduce sexual libido; epilepsy, during much of the nineteenth century, was thought to be caused by excessive masturbation, ergo, bromides that reduced sexual impulses should also reduce epileptic seizures. This event is one of many examples of how a theory that makes no sense may, nevertheless, lead to the right results.

Chloralhydrate was introduced into medical practice as a hypnotic in 1868, and it proved to be so excellently suited for this purpose that today, more than a century later, it is still one of our best hypnotics. Incidentally, chloralhydrate provides another historical example of the right result having been generated by an incorrect theory. Liebreich, who introduced chloralhydrate as a hypnotic, had done so on the theory that the drug would be metabolized in the body to chloroform and thus put the patient to sleep. Chemically, this action makes no sense. But the drug works and that is all that really matters in psychopharmacotherapy. Why it works is a question for psychopharmacology.

In 1903, Fischer and von Mering synthesized Veronal as a hypnotic barbiturate that was, together with many other barbiturates, to reign supreme for more than a generation as the remedy for insomnia. The story is that Fischer and von Mering named the drug Veronal because they had designed its formula on a train just as it pulled into the station of Verona. Today we have learned to prescribe barbiturates with greater caution than in those days because we are better informed about their limitations, toxicity, and addictive potential. But in the first third of our century the many varieties of barbiturates (several dozens were available—long-acting, intermediate, short-acting, ultra-short-acting ones) were, besides chloralhydrate, the only respectable representatives of psychopharmacotherapeutic agents.

The next pharmacological attack on psychological foes of humanity was made on inhibition-inertia, when Prinzmetal and Bloomberg in 1935 introduced the amphetamines into medicine. These drugs are powerful stimulants with some euphorizing effects, and there were high hopes in the beginning that a cure for depression had been found. It became soon evident that this hope could not be realized and that the therapeutic uses of amphetamines and amphetamine-like drugs are quite limited, although their abuses abound.

There followed a brief period, during and after World War II, when narcoanalysis was much in vogue as a psychiatric treatment modality. This technique utilized the disinhibition produced by an intravenous injection of a short-acting barbiturate, either alone or in combination with an amphetamine, to elicit otherwise suppressed information and intense emotional responses from the patient, as an adjunct to psychotherapy.

At about that time too, a major advance in psychiatric drug therapy was made when Cade in Australia discovered the *antimanic* effects of lithium. Although this turned out to be close to the first really disease-specific treatment for any psychiatric functional disorder, its significance was not fully recognized for another 15 or 20 years, perhaps, because our psychopharmacological and neurochemical knowledge of the affective disorders was still so limited at that time.

In the early 1950s came the most dramatic breakthrough in psycho-pharmacotherapy since the advent of anesthesia a century before. Delay and Deniker reported from France that a newly synthesized drug, chlorpromazine, produced an unusual state of sedation in animals and humans and had shown unexpected therapeutic effects in psychiatric patients. It soon became clear that this drug had a reliable suppressant action on *psychotic syndromes,* more specifically on such cognitive and perceptual symptoms as thought disorder, delusions, and hallucinations.

I remember how skeptical I was at first about these claims. In order to establish whether the sedative action of chlorpromazine was really qualitatively different from that of the traditional hypnotics I set up an experiment that is worth describing here briefly, as an illustration of the almost unbelievably naive way in which clinical research could still proceed only 25 years ago. I asked eight nurses to volunteer for the experiment which consisted in performing a few tests, i.e., reaction time (R.T.), tapping speed (TAP), digit span forward (D.F.), and digit symbol substitution (D.S.) before and one hour after receiving an oral dose of secobarbital (SB) and, on another day, before and one hour after an oral dose of chlorpromazine (CP) that was about equivalent to the secobarbital in its drowsiness-inducing effects. Figure 2 is

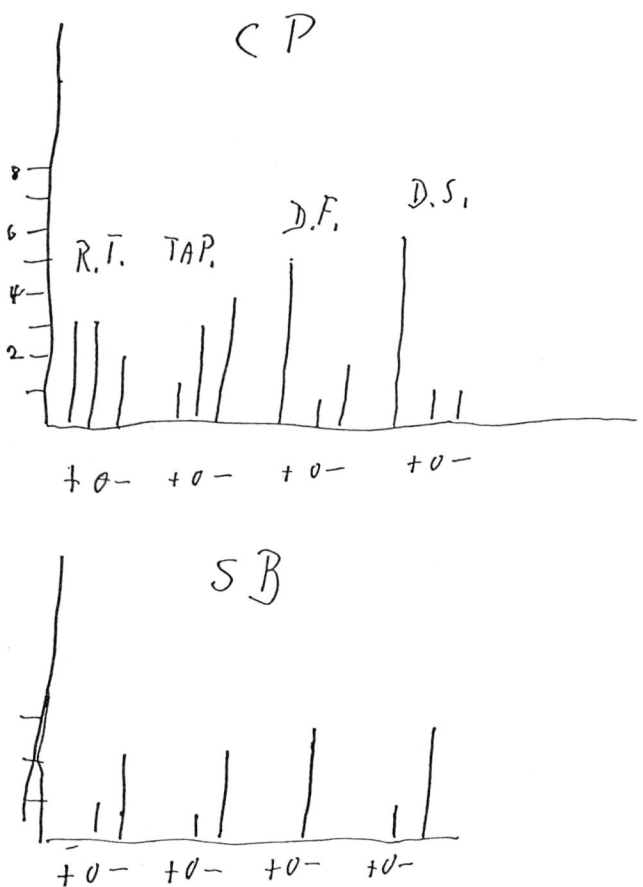

Figure 2
Original notes on the author's first experiments comparing effects
of Chlorpromazine and Secobarbital on some performance tests.

R.T.: reduction line
TAP.: taping speed
D.F.: digit forward
D.S.: digit symbol substitution

a copy of the original, roughly drawn scores of improved perform-ance (+), no change (0) and decreased performance (–). For the secobarbital condition I thought I needed only three subjects, since the results were so conspicuously different from those under chlor-promazine. My evaluation of the results was made by inspection of these graphs with no attempt at statistical tests, and I never confirmed my impression by a duplication of the experiment. Nevertheless, these results convinced me that chlorpromazine did indeed induce a new kind of sedation that seemed to be dissociated from the "dopi-ness," the impaired performance that, we thought at that time, was an inherent component of drug-induced somnolence, since in all tests some of my subjects performed actually better under the influence of chlorpromazine, but none of the three subjects, on any test, did so under secobarbital. The fact that I was right in this instance may have been a demonstration of clinical judgment, which has been defined as the ability to draw correct conclusions from insufficient evidence, or just luck. At any rate, armed with my new pharmacodynamic insight I immediately set up a clinical trial of chlorpromazine with some 70 schizophrenic patients. There were no government regula-tions, no institutional review boards, no research protocols, no formal diagnostic criteria, no double-blind procedures, no rating scales, no wash-out periods, and no need for statistical evaluation to encumber me at that time. Of course, there also was no financial support of any kind or additional personnel or equipment to help me. The results were worth the efforts in terms of work and decision-making that had gone into this trial. Weighty decisions had to be made since nobody in those days shared the responsibility of the clinical investigator, and no guidelines for procedure were available.

Other phenothiazine drugs were soon developed and tried under better controlled conditions with much the same, surprising results. But not for another year or two did psychiatrists dare to admit openly that these drugs, simple pills, were really suppressing delusions and hallucinations. I recall distinctly how apologetic I was when, at a professional meeting, I first referred to the phenothiazines as "anti-psychotic" drugs.

Then, in rapid succession, came the *antidepressants,* when Kline reported on the MAO inhibitors and, almost simultaneously, Kuhn on the tricyclics. We had some ideas how the MAO inhibitors worked but, at first, no notion of the action mechanisms of the tricyclics or, for that matter, of the antipsychotic action mechanism of the phenothiazines, at least, not for several years.

Finally, in 1960, Randall reported on the "taming" action of chlordiazepoxide (Librium) and thus introduced the benzodiazepines, the first low toxicity, minor tranquilizers into the treatment of anxiety. Many other benzodiazepine derivatives have been developed since then by industry, and quite a few are in clinical use today as hypnotics, or mainly as anxiolytic sedatives.

The history of psychopharmacotherapy terminates at this point and no major turns or steps appear on the horizon. No doubt, there will be more exciting developments in psychiatric drug therapy, but in the last few years the rapid progress of psychopharmacological research seems to have overtaken clinical psychopharmacotherapy whose last phases of therapeutic attacks on the affective disorders, the psychoses, and anxiety are far from being concluded.

Psychopharmacology: Historical Review

If we now glance briefly at the history of psychopharmacology (see Figure 3), we find that its development started with some early achievements of organic chemistry, e.g., the analytic isolation of morphine from opium by Sertürner in 1803, the production of chloralhydrate by Liebig in 1832, almost 40 years before Liebreich introduced this compound into therapeutics, and the synthesis of barbituric acid in 1864 by von Baeyer, again about 40 years before its clinical application by Fischer and von Mering.

This chemical phase of building the foundations of psychopharmacology lasted for the better part of the nineteenth century. It was followed by the first elementary experiments in psychopharmacology, conducted by Kraepelin, the father of modern psychiatry, who in Wundt's laboratory investigated the effects of various psychotropic drugs, including caffeine and alcohol, on simple mental functions. Although Kraepelin's methodology was very primitive compared to today's standards, he acquired his lasting fame in other areas of psychiatry. He nevertheless was one of the first to introduce laboratory procedures into psychopharmacology (Kraepelin, 1892).

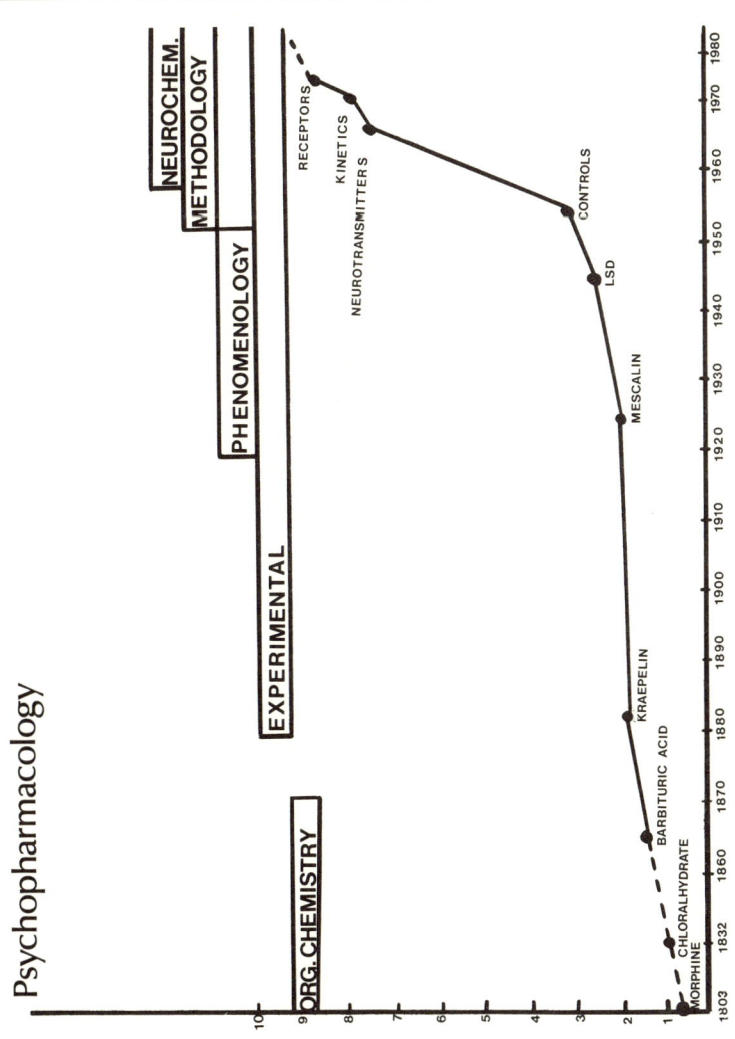

Figure 3
Historical developments in psychopharmacology and their
relative importance from 1803 to the present

There was not much further activity in the field until the 1920s and 1930s when, at the University of Heidelberg, and later at the Maudsley Clinic in London, well-designed experiments with the hallucinogenic drug mescalin were carried out. Lewin had published his basic book on hallucinogens, *Phantastica,* and there was much interest in the new and strange mental phenomena that were produced by these drugs (Lewin, 1931). These studies in *phenomenology* were crowned by Hofmann's accidental discovery of LSD and its striking effects in 1943. Here was a substance that, in incredibly small amounts, experimentally produced psychotic states in normal volunteers. This psychotomimetic action of LSD was a tremendous stimulant to neurophysiologists and neurochemists to study the action mechanisms of LSD, in the hope that they may provide valuable clues to the causes of schizophrenia.

However, the most powerful impetus to psychopharmacology came a few years later with the discovery of the antipsychotic effects of the phenothiazines and other neuroleptic drugs. For the first time in psychiatry there were now drugs with reliable, therapeutic effects in psychotic states. The immediate consequence was the almost explosive development of the *methodology* of clinical trials to assure the best possible control. That methodology meant working out techniques for double-blind procedures, constructing rating scales for more objective monitoring of patients, establishing well-defined diagnostic criteria for the selection of patients, and developing computer programs for sophisticated, statistical evaluation of the results of clinical trials.

Once set into motion, psychopharmacology this time did not stop again. The clinical discovery of the antidepressants a few years after discovery of the antipsychotics led psychopharmacologists to the elucidation of the role of neurotransmitters in the brain. That, in turn, provided fertile hypotheses on the causes of depression, the action mechanisms of antidepressants, i.e., the reestablishment of a disturbed noradrenaline-serotonin balance, and the action mechanism of antipsychotic drugs, i.e., the blocking of dopaminergic neurons. All this research was followed by a host of new findings in the fields of neurochemistry, neuroendocrinology, and neurophysiology, many of which also had an important impact on psychopharmacology: for example, the discoveries of specific receptors for opiates and benzodiazepines, followed by discovery of the endorphins and the work on other neuropeptides, as well as the mass of new information on pharmacokinetics. There is little doubt that, as of today, the scientific component of psychopharmacology is progressing more rapidly than the clinical.

The Present and Its Problems

These new and fundamental discoveries and theories on the functioning of our brain could not fail to have an impact on the whole epistemological background of the behavioral sciences. The precarious parallelism that traditionally has been the philosophical perspective in which scientists approach the mind-body problem has been powerfully modified by the recent discoveries in psychopharmacology, which will allow us today to form theories that reduce some mere associations of mental and physical phenomena to real cause-effect relationships.

Only thirty years ago, no other psychological symptoms than pain and agitation could be reliably influenced by drugs, and such complex phenomena as hallucinations, delusions, and mood disorders appeared to be beyond the range of any chemical modification or biological explanation. Because this limitation is no longer true today, many thousands of patients who had to be hospitalized before can now live in the community and be treated in outpatient clinics. These therapeutic and theoretical developments in psychopharmacology have also forged strong new links between psychiatry and the rest of medicine with its primarily biological orientation.

There are also unintended nonscientific and nontherapeutic offshoots of psychopharmacology, such as the development of a new multimillion-dollar psychopharmaceutical industry and, on the negative side, the street-drug culture of a society that, in search for new modes of altering consciousness, has made nonmedical use of the new pharmacological technology.

But, in today's psychopharmacotherapy many problems are still with us. The long-term drug treatment of psychotic patients carries a 15 to 25 percent risk of tardive dyskinesia developing as a dreaded complication. Furthermore, while antipsychotic drugs are very effective in suppressing active symptoms in acute psychotic states, they are much less effective in combating so-called negative symptoms in chronic conditions, for example, withdrawal, passivity, and inertia. Our antidepressant drugs are effective only in 60 to 65 percent of depressed patients and take a long time before showing results (2 to 3 weeks), while electroconvulsive treatment works in 85 percent of patients and often in a few days. In addition, today's antidepressants are still more toxic than would be desirable for drugs to be placed safely into the hands of potentially suicidal patients.

Paradoxically, the problems with anxiolytic drugs are mainly related to the fact that these drugs are very reliable in their symptomatic effectiveness and cause almost no immediate, adverse side effects so that patients and physicians alike are often tempted to overuse them by prescribing them too quickly and for too long a period of time, often in response to the patient's urgings. Patients also become tolerant to these drugs and then tend to increase their doses frequently without authorization. As a result, the patients may develop psychological and even physical dependence on the anxiolytic. Furthermore, it is a fact that we do not yet have any true and specific anxiolytic drug; all our anxiolytic sedatives are basically hypnotics, with more or less pronounced primary effects on the arousal system.

Possibilities for the Future

And what may we find in the years to come? Predicting the future is always a risky business, but there are certain developments in psychopharmacology that we may reasonably expect to happen (Lehmann, 1977). For instance, it is very likely that antipsychotic drugs of the future will not cause as many extrapyramidal side effects as today's neuroleptics do, and they will probably no longer carry such a heavy risk of tardive dyskinesia. Future antidepressants will be less toxic and more effective than today's MAO inhibitors and tricyclics; they will also act more rapidly. Most important, we may hope that antipsychotic and antidepressant drugs of the future will attack mental disorders at more fundamental, possibly enzymatic, levels of cerebral metabolism, not just at their final common paths, and thus will bring us closer to a real cure of schizophrenia and affective disorders.

New anxiolytic sedatives might be more specific and reduce excessive anxiety without producing drowsiness or any decrease of alertness and cognitive or psychomotor performance. They will probably combine suppression of peripheral effects of sympathetic excitation, similar to the action of specific alpha and beta blockers, with a central action on the affective component of anxiety that will block subjective dysphoria without producing disinhibition, tolerance, or dependence. Anxiolytic drugs as well as hypnotics of the future might well be some naturally occurring hypothalamic peptides.

Eventually, we may also have drugs that will regulate not only the various electroencephalographic stages of our sleep spectrum, one by one, in frequency and duration, but also our dreams, their occurrence, vividness, recall, and even, to some extent, their content with regard to bizarreness and euphoric, indifferent, or dysphoric feeling tone.

Perhaps we will develop the ideal euphoriant that would be reliable, not disorganizing like hallucinogenic drugs, not intoxicating like alcohol, and not habit-forming like the opiates. There is a real need for such a drug among the severely disabled and the aged, who have reached the point where neither medical art and science nor social intervention of any kind can offer them help or relief in their despair and isolation.

We will probably learn how to regulate the sensitivity of many receptors in the brain and increase or decrease the sensitivity according to therapeutic needs. We may acquire the capacity to mobilize dormant, adaptive, and compensatory mechanisms of the central nervous system. Perhaps we can even discover how to regenerate nerve cells and to recapture for the adult brain some of the plasticity of its foetal and early infantile stages.

Finally, I feel confident that we will make substantial progress in the further development of drugs belonging to the new class of nootropic substances that are characterized by their selective action on the highest functions of the brain, that is, on cognitive functions, such as learning and memory. Psychopathology due to organic brain disease so far has not yielded to psychopharmacological interventions. Yet, in Canada alone today, there are close to two million people over sixty years of age and, if we consider that from 6 to 10 percent of all people over sixty-five years of age manifest various degrees of dementia, there are today from 100 to 200 thousand patients in Canada and one to two million in the United States suffering from organic brain disease for which no specific therapy is available. Nootropic drugs that can correct impaired metabolism of brain cells while such impairment is still reversible might become an effective future weapon against the destructive action of aging on one of our most precious heritages, our intact mental powers.

References

Berger, F. M. Social implications of psychotropic drugs. *Advances in Pharmacology and Chemotherapy* 10: 105–118, 1972.

Brill, H., and Patton, R. E. Analysis of population reduction in New York State mental hospitals during the first four years of large-scale therapy with psychotropic drugs. *American Journal of Psychiatry* 116: 495–509, 1959.

Freud, S. *Standard Edition of the Complete Psychological Works of Sigmund Freud.* Translated and edited by James Strachey, volume 23 (an outline of psychoanalysis), chapter 6, p. 182 (the techniques of psychoanalysis). London: Hogarth Press, 1964.

Kraepelin, E. Über die beeinflussung einfacher psychischer vorgange durch einige arzneimittel, 1892.

Lehmann, H. E. Drugs of the future. *Psychotherapeutic Drugs,* Part II. Usdin/Forrest (eds.), chapter XI-2, 1469–1489, 1977.

Lewin, L. *Phantastica; Narcotic and Stimulating Drugs, Their Use and Abuse.* London: Routledge, 1931.

New Programs for a Changing Outpatient Population

Stanley J. J. Freeman, M.D., M.A., D. Psych.

While it is true that change is inevitable and ubiquitous, it is almost as though psychiatry, psychiatrists, and psychiatric patients have had a special corner on the change market for the past century. Moreover, it looks as though change will continue to be the hallmark of our guild as we move, or are swept, along with the eighties. Prognosticators on all sides foretell a wide variety of futures for us, ranging from our growth in numbers and influence to our steady attrition and ultimate professional demise. In this paper I examine some of the more obvious and inevitable of the upcoming changes in our patients and in our practice.

As you will see, many of the proposed solutions to our problems are known and implementable today. I would venture to say that if we were to make no new discoveries in the eighties; if we were, instead, to devote all our efforts to developing programs that made use of the portion of our knowledge that is well established, it would be a decade well spent.

With a view to identifying resistance before content, let us look, first of all, at why we have not narrowed the gap between what is known and what is applied. The factors opposing this narrowing are elements of the same resistance that, unless dealt with, will also prevent an imaginative approach to the new problems of the next ten years. This resistance originated in part, from the strong psychoanalytic influence that followed the Second World War. Of whatever persuasion, psychotherapy became a highly valued skill. The fantasy that attracted most of us into our profession had us sitting one-to-one with a patient on whom we lavished our acceptance, our beneficence, and our remarkable ability to unravel his/her tangled experiences and to repackage them into health-promoting metaphors. To be sure, we made strides in group therapy, family therapy, hypnotherapy, behavior therapy, community intervention, and all sorts of other innovative programs. But always some kind of inertial system, some invisible gyroscope, kept bringing us back to our central activity, one-to-one psychotherapy. Despite all our efforts to the contrary, we kept selecting for our caseloads "good" patients; that is, those who were psychologically minded and had the kinds of conflict neuroses we had studied in our training.

Before we blame all of this "inertia" on psychoanalysis, which, needless to say, was a crucial and beneficial influence in other ways, let us also remember another factor that shaped our practice. In this century, the word "acute" confers more status than the word "chronic"; and the word "cure," a great deal more than "palliation" or "support." This status is as true for general medicine as it is for psychiatry. Every one of us has started at least one program for chronic psychotics, persons with severe personality disorders, the noncopers, or the alcohol-abusers, but such programs have a half-life of about two years. What stays constant is "regular" psychotherapy with good-prognosis neurotics.

Clearly, then, in order to tend to some of the necessary tasks, we need psychiatrists who can think in terms of therapeutic and community systems, who can see that real status comes from dealing with the most difficult patients, and who know enough about program development to take a leadership role in applying what is known to the solution of both the well entrenched and the newly developing problems.

This argument probably sounds familiar. We heard some of the same arguments back in the sixties when the community psychiatry movement began. We read about it in Caplan's books (18, 19). Many of us looked to the community mental health centers (CMHCs) to take care of this aspect of things and, to some extent, they did. But the old gyroscope kept nudging the psychiatrists back to psychotherapy and turning the CMHCs over to other mental health professionals. Winslow (105) provides some telling data to illustrate this point. In 1970 there were 3.1 full-time psychiatrists per CMHC; by 1975 this figure had dropped to 2.4. From 1970 to 1975 the number of CMHCs increased over 100 percent, while full-time equivalent psychiatrists increased only 50 percent, social workers 150 percent, and psychologists 250 percent. I have no doubt that in outpatient centers of general hospitals, psychiatric hospitals, and university clinics, the programs delivering some of the same services as CMHCs showed a similar trend.

Is this occurrence necessarily bad? I think it is—both from the point of view of the patient and the psychiatrist. In the case of the latter, he/she could become an endangered species. Other nonpsychiatric therapists are performing psychotherapy (by any other name) very well. There is an increasing chance that psychopharmacology may soon be quite amenable to practice by other medical practitioners. If psychiatrists bow out of mental health programming, what is left for them but gradual eclipse? If such were to occur, I think the patient would be the loser. In a time of specialization and compartmentalization of professional expertise, there is a great need for a central switching point in the system that is grounded in all of medicine, psychology, and sociology. It is at this central point that assessment, referral, and coordination of services occur at the level of the individual patient. This point is also the locus of program planning and development for the mental health system. The only logical candidate to fill this position is the psychiatrist whose training comes closest—and could easily come closer—to this ideal.

Where shall we get this psychiatrist—one who is grounded in medicine, psychology, and sociology; trained to plan, to consult, to supervise; endowed with the aura of credibility; and skilled in eliciting cooperation and enthusiasm from co-workers? I would maintain that to answer this question is the most important challenge facing educators in psychiatry today. We shall need role models, training settings, and new funds for pilot projects in which to involve our trainees. Winslow's data (105) do not augur well for our ability to involve psychiatric residents in such programs. He points out that there has been a drop in the number of psychiatrists receiving part of their training in CMHCs: 2.4 per CMHC in 1970 compared to 1.1. per CMHC in 1975. Over the same period psychology trainees increased from 0.8 to 1.7 and social work trainees from 1.4 to 2.2. Meanwhile, the caseload of the CMHCs increased by 50 percent, including a large percentage of former inpatients with major mental disorders.

There is a vicious circle in operation here. New programs for problem populations do not get started, or are not maintained, unless they are seen as high status activities by the staff. We cannot develop psychiatric staff with this orientation as long as the theoreticians and teachers regard it as hack work. Furthermore, even if the universities came to see program developers as an elite group, they would have difficulty finding training placements where the necessary skills could be learned in an environment of professional excitement and pride.

Having glanced briefly at some of the reasons for the excessive lag between psychiatric knowledge and practice, and having cast a puzzled and rather unproductive glance at possible remedies, we now consider some of the challenges that lie before us in the eighties.

Implementing What We Already Know

Post-Hospital Follow-up Programs

Aftercare of the psychotic patient remains one of the pressing problems in psychiatric case management (68, 48, 11, 6, 37, 95). A few court actions have even established a "right to aftercare" (74). Nevertheless, the deplorable conditions under which some patients are forced to live in the name of deinstitutionalization have caused an upsurge of pressure to resume long-term hospitalization. There is an impressive amount of evidence that well-conceived aftercare programs can keep patients out of the hospital and can do so with a quality of life that is more comfortable, less psychopathogenic, and more in keeping with the human dignity that we would want for them (4). We know that housing with graded supervision (85, 33, 32), social/recreational facilities (33, 1, 13), vocational training opportunities (90, 75, 29), home-visiting programs (16, 17, 46, 47, 67), training in life skills (12, 43, 41, 36, 4, 6), and, above all, proper follow-up (4, 5, 62, 49) can augment the undoubtedly strong effect of neuroleptic medication in keeping patients functioning at their best levels. To this list we should probably add patient groups that encourage self-regulation of medication (40) and support for the families of patients, including "patient sitters," homemaking services, and support groups (10). Special attention should be drawn to Anthony's work on the training of rehabilitation therapists (4).

It is worth considering for a moment where such aftercare programs should be centered. By and large, follow-up programs operated by inpatient departments have not done well. Outpatient departments attached to hospitals have, similarly, not provided the necessary spectrum of services, for some of the reasons already postulated. Indeed, a survey in which we are presently engaged (of 750 patients discharged from four hospitals) is rapidly leading us to the belief that discharge planning, follow-up, and rehabilitation would best be completely disconnected from the hospitals. The staff of a separate rehabilitation clinic or agency would be able to maintain the attitudinal set necessary to help a patient adapt to the community. They would be able to devote all of their energy and time to coordinate, or even operate, the necessary community facilities. Even the back-up psychiatrist in such a clinic would be from the community rather than the hospital. In short, what I have suggested is a new, specialized outpatient center based on the synthesis of a number of already well-established concepts and programs.

Intervention in Transitional Crises

Since Lindemann's studies of the families of victims of the Coconut Grove fire (56), there has been a growing interest in the impact of developmental transitions and stressful life events (whether sudden or ongoing) on individuals and families. The literature is voluminous and excellent reviews have appeared on many aspects of the subject (for example, 59, 65, 76, 77, 78, 96, 101). Recently the subject has taken an exciting direction with the demonstration that there is a relationship between life stress and certain changes in the immune system (83). This relationship may well foreshadow a new understanding of the mechanisms that "transduce" emotion into somatic manifestations.

The fact that mental, emotional, social, and physical dysfunction was shown to be associated with life stress soon led to a number of apparently successful interventions, both preventive and therapeutic (79, 80, 81, 82, 91, 98, 104). In general, these interventions have involved some way of identifying the group at risk, followed by the application of various forms of social support (21) and including cognitive "road maps" of what to expect and how to handle it (103), opportunities to express and to work through affect (88), and practical assistance.

Again, the physical location of programs of this sort is of interest. Some of them, such as marital separation groups, are conveniently located in the clinic setting. Others, such as programs with new cancer patients, will take place in the hospital wards under the direction of consultation-liaison teams. Of greater interest are the models in which mental health teams might travel with the police or the coroner (23, 51, 106); where liaisons with industry might be established to deal with alcoholism problems (87) or with executives recovering from myocardial infarction; where ongoing community support is given to self-help groups (for example, a multiple sclerosis association) in their own headquarters. The mobile team, modeled after the consultation-liaison team, which goes out from the outpatient clinic to a satellite, to another agency, or to the patient's home, is a therapeutic modality whose usefulness is just beginning to be recognized, and it will be discussed later.

Despite the excellent models available, few outpatient centers have made such interventions a standard part of their ongoing programming. An enthusiasm for program development is a prerequisite for such projects and we have deplored already its lack in our ranks. Therefore, newly bereaved parents, children, and spouses continue to walk out of the hospital unattended. Young men with amputations still receive physical treatment without attention to their psychic pain. Patients are still not helped to live with—or to die from—life-threatening illnesses. Clearly, this situation must change and, in fact, *is* changing. I predict that outpatient centers will achieve a great deal in this area of programming in the eighties.

Changes in Societal Expectations, Values and Mores

The Psychiatrist as "Doctor of Happiness"

The term "neurosis" has acquired a broad connotation of non-organic personal distress that does not interfere with reality and includes the classical symptom neuroses, the personality disorders characterized by aberrant overall lifestyles, and a vague assortment of behavior patterns that restrict relationships with others. In addition, one must include those who seek psychiatric help for loneliness, despair, unhappiness, lack of fulfillment, or an uncertainty in personal identity (20). Our outpatient centers have more than doubled their number of treatment episodes since 1955 (11), and the greatest number of the patients have been labeled neurotic. There has been a corresponding increase of inpatient admissions for so-called neurotics (61).

Chodoff (20) who coined the term "Doctor of Happiness," used as the heading for this section, accounts for this increase, not as a greater vulnerability to neurosis but rather as "a readiness to label as neurotic forms of personal discomfort and maladaptive behavior that previously would have been considered within the bounds of normal." We are all, it appears, *entitled* to happiness, or if not happiness, at least to freedom from discomfort. What was once a "natural" reaction to a distressing event or life condition has now become a symptom or even an illness. And it is the psychiatrist, the "Doctor of Happiness," who is called upon to bring the sufferer to his rightful state of contentment, if not, euphoria.

This trend has two important consequences. In the first place, it is imperative that we recognize our too frequent acquiescence to the demand that we assuage all pain and discomfort; we also need to help our patients work through their crises in growth-promoting ways. Much has been written about the excessive use of the minor tranquilizers. Every year, in both Canada and the United States, one person in five gets a prescription for anti-anxiety medication (63). Fejer and Smart showed that in just three years (between 1971 and 1974) the use of tranquilizers in Metropolitan Toronto increased dramatically from 12.79 to 19.0 percent of the population (31). I believe that psychiatric workers have already become alarmed at this trend and will take a leadership role in educating other physicians to limit sharply their use of the minor psychoactive drugs.

The second consequence of the predilection of society to turn to us for the relief of all psychic discomfort is the necessity to learn and to teach techniques for helping a new population of patients. It has already been mentioned that we are learning a good deal about populations going through situational and developmental stress reactions and that many useful intervention techniques are being developed to help them. Similarly, many researchers are looking at the differential effectiveness of various coping styles with new interest (3, 73, 100).

Meanwhile, despite the fact that these more widely defined neurotics now outnumber the conflict neurotics in our outpatient centers, and despite the fact that adequate techniques are being developed to deal with some of them, we still practice and teach that old-time religion: traumatic early experience must be de-repressed. If that is not possible, administer "supportive" therapy (for which read, give medication for symptoms and see them as infrequently as possible). I suggest that a very important priority for the eighties is that we teach ourselves and our students how to intervene in a crisis, how to realign a social support system, how to teach more effective relational and problem-solving skills, and, of course, how to determine which patients need these interventions. The enthusiasm for program development that I extolled earlier is, needless to say, highly relevant.

Women as Psychiatric Patients

The topic of women as patients, and particularly as psychiatric patients, has received considerable attention in the past decade (92, 26, 42). It has long been observed that women with nonpsychotic psychiatric disorders are over-represented in outpatient centers. They have been shown to have higher rates of neurotic illness than men, more symptoms of physical and mental discomfort, and a greater tendency to health-seeking behavior (24). Even more ominously, they outnumber men more than two to one in their use of prescription psychotropic drugs (24, 25, 31). In fact, in Fejer and Smart's Toronto study, the use of minor tranquilizers by women rose from 16.3 percent in 1971 to 25.2 percent in 1974. In the same period the rates for men remained the same.

A common explanation for increased usage of tranquilizers by women is that there is increasing role strain, role overload, and role ambiguity among women. It is simply too difficult, the argument goes, to be wife, mother, and member of the work force. However, there is evidence to the contrary. Guse and colleagues (39) found that working women reported lower psychotropic drug use than women who were full-time homemakers. There was, in fact, a significant negative correlation between the amount of time spent working outside the home and drug use.

Lest I give the impression that work will be the salvation of womankind, let me hasten to acknowledge the obvious: we are dealing with a complex, multifactorial problem. But one of the factors seems to be that many psychiatrists have tended to reflect the traditional assumption that a discontented homemaker is either bad or sick. In our case, "sick" is the operative concept and we have tended to "treat" them. I think this situation has begun to shift in the past five years, and I would predict major changes in both conceptualization and practice in the eighties. It is a fairly safe prediction. Our female colleagues in psychiatry give every indication of not allowing us to drag our feet.

Changes in the Structure of the Family

We continue to talk of "the family" as though it were the structure we grew up with. We take its permanence and values as given. In fact, such families are now in the minority in North America; only 16 percent of U.S. households have the traditional pattern of working father and full-time homemaker mother. Approximately 50 percent of women are in the work force and one-third of mothers with children under age three have jobs outside the home. By the end of the eighties, one out of every three children will have lived at one time with a divorced parent. Ten percent of Canadian babies (16 percent in the United States) are born to unmarried mothers (34).

As a profession we have not addressed the implications of these trends adequately for both theory and practice. We have yet to study how a working mother and a day-care center alter the developmental stages of the child. We need to know what happens to the metapsychology, which was originally based on the father-mother-child triad, when "father" (who is not father but mother's new spouse), the biological father (and his new wife), and four sets of "grandparents" are still very much in the picture.

Although several models exist (89), outpatient centers have not yet made pre-marriage schools or, better still, one-year-after-marriage schools part of their regular programming. Marital counseling services and support groups for separated couples are fairly common but there are still very few programs to help the remarried and their reconstituted families with the special problems to which they are vulnerable (64, 99).

It seems to me, from the vantage point of the beginning of the decade, that investigation in this area will be as important as intervention. We simply have to find out what it all means and what its consequences are before we are in a position to design and implement relevant therapeutic procedures.

New Patient Populations for the 1980s

Some of the patient populations that will demand more of our attention in the 1980s will do so because they are increasing rapidly in numbers, for example, the elderly. Others will do so because society is at last recognizing that they have been cut off from mainstream services by barriers of language, culture, social class, economic insolvency, bilateral prejudice, and maldistribution of psychiatric services. Among these groups are the Indians and the Inuit, the minority groups (particularly the "visible minorities"), large segments of the economically depressed, immigrant groups, and those who reside in the sparsely populated regions of the continent. I shall mention three of these population groups—native Indians and Inuit, the elderly, and immigrants.

Native Indians and Inuit

In this section I shall deal with the native population living on the reserves and in the Arctic. It is admitted that the native population of this continent has been robbed systematically of its land, its culture, its heritage, and its dignity. Only now are some of them beginning to look at themselves as a people with a tradition worthy of pride. Leighton (52) has pointed out that in any society where organization and institutions have been destroyed the prevalence of psychiatric impairment (emotional, mental, and behavioral) is increased. This occurrence has been the case in many native communities, and it points the way to amelioration of the situation. Clearly the native peoples must be given the opportunity to take control of their lives and to regain their former pride. These are the prerequisites of the kind of societal organization that Leighton has demonstrated to be associated with mental health.

If the first move for clinicians is to provide conventional clinical services for the casualties of the current system, we must make as much use as possible of native health aides and even native healers. The goal would be to turn the leadership of our programs over to the natives as quickly as possible and to provide services according to priorities they set.

In case you are wondering about the relevance of this discussion to psychiatric outpatient centers, it is this: it has proved almost impossible to attract psychiatrists to sparsely populated areas. In the few successful programs, traveling psychiatrists have provided consultation and backup to mental health professionals living in the area. They, in turn, give some direct service to clients, help local professionals (physicians, welfare workers, etc.) with their cases, and coordinate access to the visiting psychiatrist. Two successful examples of this model originate from the University of Toronto; one to the Indians of northwestern Ontario (98) and one to the Inuit of the eastern Arctic (8, 9). It is my belief that this form of outreach model has wide application. Similar programs for special populations, whether located close by or at a distance, should be part of the total program of most outpatient centers.

Psychiatric Services for the Elderly

It has become almost tiresome to be reminded that the proportion of elderly persons in the population is increasing rapidly. Yet, it is a fact, and one that must compel our attention. By 2001, 12 percent of Canadians will be over 65 and their numbers will have risen from 1.8 million to 3.3 million (86). In the United States the comparable figure for 2001 will be 28 million individuals over the age of 65 (70). The elderly are also the age group most susceptible to mental illness. The incidence of psychiatric disorder rises from 76.3 per 100,000 for ages

25 to 34 to 235.1 per 100,000 for ages 65 and over (15). The prevalence rates are, of course, much higher.

Despite the high incidence of psychiatric disorder and the growing evidence that good response to treatment is by no means infrequent, the elderly, as a group, are underrepresented in private psychiatric practice and in outpatient facilities of general hospitals and community mental health centers (22). At the same time, they are overrepresented in inpatient facilities, especially in state hospitals (84). The unfavorable ratio between inpatient and outpatient utilization is, of course, reflective of the mistakenly hopeless prognosis still assigned to the elderly. The trend toward institutionalization is also seen in the heavy use of homes for the aged and nursing homes. In Ontario 9.2 percent of persons over 65 are in institutions compared to 4.5 percent in Britain (86).

There are a number of reasons for this difference. In the first place, the recent increase in attention to the diagnostic assessment of the elderly has demonstrated that a large number of functional (usually treatable) illnesses have been misdiagnosed as organic brain syndromes (27, 102). Such misdiagnosis seems to be more true for North America than for Europe. Secondly, factors such as climate, geography, population mobility, and family style clearly differentiate England from Ontario. Perhaps the most important factor is that home care services in Canada were not insured simultaneously with hospital and institutional care, as they were in Britain (86). (Let the United States take note of this point as it develops health insurance programs.)

The negatives associated with institutionalization of the elderly have been summarized by Lieberman (53). They include increased mortality and morbidity, impairment of memory, poor performance on perceptual functioning tests, increased depression, and lowered morale and life satisfaction. Even though many of the studies demonstrating these effects have been strongly criticized by Kasl (45), we would all agree that unneccessary institutionalization is to be avoided at all costs. Aside from its potentially deleterious physical and psychiatric sequelae, it commits the patient to a lifestyle without dignity, self-determination, or self-respect.

We must, therefore, be vigorous advocates of the development of strong support systems for the elderly, including health care, social service, housing, recreation, education, transportation, and volunteer services. If well designed, these systems can markedly increase the quality and duration of non-institutional living.

As to clinical services in 1971, the Committee on Aging of the Group for the Advancement of Psychiatry (GAP) laid down a set of very sound principles for delivering psychiatric services to the elderly—principles that countered regressive tendencies in patients and maximized participation of all the helping personnel involved (38). Reduced to its simplest terms, the Report advocated that the consultants go to the patients wherever they lived, rather than bring the patients into a special unit. In this way they could work with families or nursing home staff helping them to maintain the psychogeriatric patients where they were.

It is remarkable that ten years later, the GAP recommendations have still not achieved widespread implementation. This lack will undoubtedly change. The number of geriatric patients is growing quickly even as the funding for expensive institutional settings is shrinking.

Psychiatric Services for Immigrant Groups

As we all know, immigration into both the United States and Canada has been very heavy since 1946. Canada alone has received over three and a half million immigrants. Within the past decade, new streams of refugees have again been created by world events. For example, two separate waves of immigration have come from southeast Asia and, recently there has been an influx from Cuba into Florida.

Depending on which study is consulted, the incidence of mental disorder in immigrants, as compared to native-born individuals, has either been equal (50), higher in immigrants (60, 71), or higher in the native born (69, 94). The differences are clearly due to the multiplicity of factors determining hospitalization, which is generally used to define mental illness. But, no matter what the differences in final outcome may be, it is clear that distress and disorganization tend to be very high among immigrants and that a variety of support measures can help ease the distress of this life event (2, 14, 54).

It is, paradoxically, within the context of greater need that we find a striking under-utilization of mental health facilities by almost all immigrant groups (2, 66). To be more exact, where there is a marked difference in culture or language, and therefore need is at its greatest, the under-utilization of services is most marked. Among the obvious reasons for this are concern for the family's immigration status, cultural differences in the meaning of mental illness, language barriers, limited knowledge about potential sources of help, and a view that emotional support and psychotherapy are not really proper forms of help (55).

The usual solution proposed by each immigrant group is an outpatient center and a hospital ward dedicated to that ethnic group and staffed by personnel grounded in their language and culture. This solution is obviously not possible given the number of ethnic groups and dearth of space, funding, and qualified staff. But other solutions should be possible. We have recently developed a proposal for a multi-ethnic agency in which teams of a particular ethnic origin, modeled on psychiatric consultation-liaison teams in general hospitals, go at scheduled times or on demand to an outpatient center, a hospital, or a community agency. There they work with the staff facilitating entry into, or exit from, the psychiatric system of members of their own ethnic group.

Whatever models will eventually emerge as most useful, it is clear that this is an area of vital concern, and one that will likely be aggravated through the eighties, given the instability of the world situation.

Changes Due to New Technology

Technological breakthroughs frequently bring about rapid progress in therapeutic techniques and in research. For example, in the past decade we have seen how the discovery of depot neuroleptics like fluphenazine enanthate led to a radical change in aftercare programs for chronic schizophrenics. The "moditen clinic" quickly became the locus for follow-up, patient clubs, and other therapeutic modalities.

I should like to discuss one technological advance that seems very promising at the present time. Interactive television (IATV) appears to be a way of delivering the psychiatrist to remote locations in a way that saves time and expense (28, 30, 72, 93). The "remote" location may be thousands of miles away and available only by satellite or it may be a nearby nursing home or a storefront clinic in a depressed area of the city. In 1978 Elton and Carey (30) reviewed twenty U.S. programs utilizing IATV.

In addition to its use as a means of providing assessment, treatment-planning, and follow-up of actual cases and their families, the system has other potential functions. Subspecialty expertise (for example, forensic) could be made available to a community in which there are simply not enough cases to warrant regular travel by an expert. Support and training could be provided for professionals and para-professionals in the remote community. Public education and organizational meetings could be carried out by IATV. Research collaboration, especially if combined with computer linkage, could greatly extend the range and variety of research projects.

Interactive television gives promise of solving many of the problems related to maldistribution of expert personnel. For example, in the programs for native peoples discussed above, the visiting psychiatrist could come weekly by IATV rather than quarterly by plane. The increased frequency would also make it possible for the psychiatrist to participate in other, less clinical activities. The Departments of Psychiatry at both the University of Toronto and the University of Western Ontario are presently exploring IATV as a way of servicing the vast areas of this province.

The Extended Consultation-Liaison Model

I should like, finally, to draw your attention once more to a program model that has been mentioned again and again in this paper. It is an extension of the typical consultation-liaison model that departments of psychiatry have developed in general hospitals all over the United States and Canada (44, 57). In this model a consultant psychiatrist typically goes to one of the hospital wards to provide consultation and treatment-planning. His/her team then works with the staff of the remote service to help them implement the psychiatrist's recommendations through education, role-modeling and interpretation.

I have suggested a very similar model for working with agencies around rehabilitation problems, for providing support to stressed populations, for breaching the language and culture barrier in immigrant groups, for providing service to sparsely settled areas, and so on. It is a powerful model and less expensive than many of its alternatives. If the very considerable costs of IATV can be brought down (there is some indication that they can), the logistics of "delivering" the consultant to his or her consultees will become much simpler.

Summary

To summarize, I have tried in this paper to draw attention to the challenges that the eighties will bring to psychiatry. Many of the special populations to whom we shall have to attend, can be well served by programs using an extension of the consultation-liaison model. Several examples of its application are given, including the use of interactive television.

It is suggested that a major resistance to effective action in both the past and the future is to be found in the fact that we have selected and trained our residents to be psychotherapists and have shown little respect for, or interest in, program development as a subspecialty in its own right.

References

1. Allodi, F., Belyea, M., Sniderman, S., & Freeman, S. J. J. The community group program: Evaluation of a multi-agency therapeutic social club. *Canadian Psychiatric Association Journal* 17: Special Supplement I, 45–50, 1972.

2. Allodi, R. The Italians of Toronto: The mental health problems of an immigrant community. In W. E. Mann (ed.), *Social Deviance in Canada*. Toronto: Copp, Clark, 1971.

3. Andrews, G., Tennant, C., Hewson, D. M., & Vaillant, G. E. Life event stress, social support, coping style, and risk of psychological impairment. *Journal of Nervous and Mental Disease* 166: 307–316, 1978.

4. Anthony, W. A., Cohen, M. R., & Vitalo, R. The measurement of rehabilitation outcome. *Schizophrenia Bulletin* 4: 365–383, 1978.

5. Anthony, W. A., Buell, G. J., Sharratt, S., & Althoff, M. E. The efficacy of psychiatric rehabilitation. *Psychological Bulletin* 78: 447–456, 1972.

6. Anthony, W. A. & Margules, A. Toward improving the efficacy of psychiatric rehabilitation: A skills training approach. *Rehabilitation Psychology* 21: 101–105, 1974.

7. Armstrong, H. Providing psychiatric care and consultation in remote Indian villages. *Hospital and Community Psychiatry* 29: 678–680, 1978.

8. Atcheson, J. D., & Malcolmson, S. A. Psychiatric consultation to the eastern Canadian Arctic communities. Proceedings of the Third International Symposium, Yellowknife, NW I. In R. J. Shepard & S. Ioth (eds.), *Circumpolar Health*, pp. 539–542. Toronto: University of Toronto Press, 1976.

9. Atcheson, J. D. Northern consultation: Problems of mental health in the Canadian Arctic. *Canada's Mental Health* 20: 10–17, 1972.

10. Atwood, N., & Williams, M. E. Group support for families of the mentally ill. *Schizophrenia Bulletin* 4: 415–425, 1978.

11. Bassuk, E., & Gerson, S. Deinstitutionalization and mental health services. *Scientific American* 238: 46–53, 1978.

12. Becker, P., & Bayer, C. Preparing chronic patients for community placement: A four-stage treatment program. *Hospital and Community Psychiatry* 26: 448–450, 1975.

13. Bill, A. Z. Social clubs help prevent readmission. *Hospital and Community Psychiatry* 21: 161–162, 1970.

14. Bourne, P. G. The Chinese students—acculturation and mental illness. *Psychiatry* 38: 269–277, 1975.

15. Butler, R. M. Psychiatry and the elderly: An overview. *American Journal of Psychiatry* 132: 893–900, 1975.

16. Campbell, W., Godfrey, M., Peace, S., Quinn, B., & Rasminsky, K. Community Occupational Therapy Associates: A model for community occupational therapy. *Canadian Journal of Occupational Therapy* 42: (4), 155–156, 1975.

17. Campbell, W. & Goldenberg, K. Model for community occupational therapy. Paper presented at World Federation of Occupational Therapy, Israel, 1978.

18. Caplan, G. *Principles of Preventive Psychiatry,* New York: Basic Books, 1964.

19. Caplan, G. *The Theory and Practice of Mental Health Consultation.* New York: Basic Books, 1970.

20. Chodoff, P. Changing styles in the neuroses. *American Journal of Psychiatry* 130: 149–151, 1973.

21. Cobb, S. Social support as a moderator of life stress. *Psychosomatic Medicine* 38: 300–314, 1976.

22. Cohen, G. Mental health services and the elderly: Needs and options. *American Journal of Psychiatry* 133: (1), 65–68, 1976.

23. Cohen, R., Sprafkin, R. P., Ogelsky, S., & Claiborn, W. L. (eds.). *Working with Police Agencies.* New York: Human Sciences Press, 1976.

24. Cooperstock, R. Psychotropic drug use among women. *Canadian Medical Association Journal* 115: 760–763, 1976.

25. Cooperstock, R. A review of women's psychotropic drug use. *Canadian Journal of Psychiatry* 24: 29–34, 1979.

26. D'Arcy, C., & Schmitz, J. A. Sex differences in the utilization of health services for psychiatric problems in Saskatchewan. *Canadian Journal of Psychiatry* 24: 19–27, 1979.

27. Duckworth, G. S. Studies of diagnosis and outcome in geropsychiatric and chronic psychiatric patients. Ph.D. thesis, University of Toronto, 1980.

28. Dwyer, T. F. Telepsychiatry: Psychiatric consultation by interactive television. *American Journal of Psychiatry* 130: 865–869, 1973.

29. Early, O., & Magnus, R. V. Industrial therapy organization (Bristol) 1960–65. *British Journal of Psychiatry* 114: 335–336, 1968.

30. Elton, M., & Carey, J. *Interactive Telecommunication Systems: A Working Paper on Implementation Problems.* New York: Alternate Media Center, New York University, 1978.

31. Fejer, D., & Smart, R. G. Changes in psychoactive drug use among adults in Metropolitan Toronto, 1971–1974. *Canada's Mental Health* 23: 6–7, 1975.

32. Fischer, L., & Freeman, S. J. J. Community resources consultants: An experimental approach to aftercare. *Canada's Mental Health* 24: 33–37, 1976.

33. Freeman, S. J. J., Fischer, L., & Sheldon, A. An agency model for developing and coordinating psychiatric aftercare. *Hospital and Community Psychiatry,* 1980.

34. Friedan, Betty. Presentation to Conference on the Future of the Family, sponsored by Washington Journalism Center, Washington D.C., February 11–14, 1980.

35. Glasscote, R. M., Cumming, E., Rutman, L. D., Susser, J. N., & Glassman, S. D. *Rehabilitating the Mentally Ill in the Community: A Study of Psychosocial Rehabilitation Centers,* pp. 41–63. Washington, D.C.: American Psychiatric Association and the National Association for Mental Health, 1971.

36. Goldstein, A. P., Sprafken, R. P., & Gershaw, N. J. *Skill Training for Community Living.* New York: Pergamon Press, 1976.

37. Group for the Advancement of Psychiatry Report. The chronic mental patient in the community. *Group for the Advancement of Psychiatry* 10: May 1978.

38. Group for the Advancement of Psychiatry, Committee on Aging. *The Aged and Community Mental Health* (Vol. VIII, Report no. 81), 1971.

39. Guse, L., Morier, G., & Ludwig, J. Winnipeg survey of prescription (mood-altering) use among women. *Technical Report, NMUDD.* Manitoba Alcoholism Foundation, October 1976.

40. Hansell, N. Services for schizophrenics: A lifelong approach to treatment. *Hospital and Community Psychiatry* 29: 105–109, 1978.

41. Hogarty, G. E., Goldberg, S., & Schooler, N. R. Drug and sociotherapy in the aftercare of schizophrenic patients. *Archives of General Psychiatry* 31: 603–608, 1974.

42. Horwitz, A. The pathways into psychiatric treatment: Some differences between men and women. *Journal of Health and Social Behavior* 18: 169–178, 1977.

43. Jacobs, M. K., & Trick, O. L. Successful psychiatric rehabilitation using an in-patient teaching laboratory. *American Journal of Psychiatry* 131: 145–148, 1974.

44. Karasu, T. B., Plutchick, R., Steinmuller, R. I., Conte, H., & Siegel, B. Patterns of psychiatric consultation in a general hospital. *Hospital and Community Psychiatry* 28: (4), 291–294, 1977.

45. Kasl, S. V. Physical and mental health effects of involuntary relocation and institutionalization on the elderly—A review. *American Journal of Public Health* 62: (3), 377, 1972.

46. Katkin, S., Ginsburg, M., Rifken, M. H., & Scott, J. T. Effectiveness of female volunteers in the treatment of outpatients. *Journal of Counseling Psychology* 18: 97–100, 1971.

47. Katkin, S., Zimmerman, V., Rosenthal, J., & Ginsburg, M. Using volunteer therapists to reduce hospital readmissions. *Hospital and Community Psychiatry* 26: 151–153, 1975.

48. Kedward, H. B., Eastwood, M. R., Allodi, R., & Duckworth, G. S. The evaluation of chronic psychiatric care. *Canadian Medical Association Journal* 110: 519–523, 1974.

49. Kirk, S. A. Effectiveness of community services for discharged mental hospital patients. *American Journal of Orthopsychiatry* 46: 646–659, 1976.

50. Krupenski, J., & Stoller, A. Incidence of mental disorders in Victoria, Australia according to the country of birth. *Medical Journal of Australia* 2: 265–279, 1965.

51. The Law Reform Commission of Canada. *Studies on Diversion.* Ottawa: Information Canada, 1975.

52. Leighton, D. C., Harding, J. S., Macklin, D. B., MacMillan, A. M., & Leighton, A. H. *The Character of Danger.* New York: Basic Books, 1963.

53. Lieberman, M. A. Institutionalization of the aged: Effects on behavior. *Journal of Gerontology* 24: 330, 1969.

54. Lin, T. Y., & Lin, M. C. Service delivery issues in Asian-North American communities. *American Journal of Psychiatry* 135: (4), 454–456, 1978.

55. Lin, T. Y., Tardiff, K., Donetz, G., & Goresky, W. Ethnicity and patterns of help-seeking. *Culture, Medicine and Psychiatry* 2: 4–13, 1978.

56. Lindemann, E. Symptomatology and management of acute grief. *American Journal of Psychiatry* 101: 141–148, 1944.

57. Lipowski, Z. J. Consultation-liaison psychiatry: An overview. *American Journal of Psychiatry* 131: 623–630, 1974.

58. Lynch, A. Report of the Committee on Mental Health Services in Ontario, p. 227. Toronto: Ontario Council of Health, 1979.

59. Macbride, A. Retirement as a life crisis: Myth or reality? A review. *Canadian Psychiatric Association Journal* 21: 547–556, 1976.

60. Malzberg, B., & Lee, E. S. *Migration and Mental Disease.* New York: Social Science Research Council, 1956.

61. Martin, B. A., Kedward, H. B., & Eastwood, M. R. Hospitalization for mental illness: Evaluation of admission trends from 1941 to 1971. *Canadian Medical Association Journal* 115: 322–325, 1976.

62. McCranie, E. W., & Mizell, T. A. Aftercare for psychiatric patients: Does it prevent rehospitalization. *Hospital and Community Psychiatry* 29: 584–587, 1978.

63. Menuck, M. Unwanted effects of Benzodiazepine tranquillizers. *Modern Medicine of Canada* 34: (12), 1637–1640, 1979.

64. Messinger, L. Remarriage between divorced people with children from previous marriages: A proposal for preparation for remarriage. *Journal of Marriage and Family Counseling* 2: (2), 193–200, 1976.

65. Minter, R. E. & Kimball, C. P. Life events and illness onset: A review. *Psychosomatics* 19: 334–339, 1978.

66. Morgan, P., & Andrushko, E. The use of diagnostic-specific rates of mental hospitalization to estimate under-utilization by immigrants. *Social Science and Medicine* 11: 611–618, 1977.

67. Mosher, L. R., Menn, A., & Matthews, S. Soteria: Evaluation of a home based treatment for schizophrenia. *American Journal of Orthopsychiatry* 45: 455–469, 1975.

68. Murphy, H. B. M. Foster homes: The new back wards? *Canada's Mental Health* 20: Supplement 71, 1972.

69. Murphy, H. B. M. Migration and the major mental disorders: A reappraisal. In M. B. Kandor (ed.), *Morbidity and Mental Health,* pp. 5–29. Springfield: Charles A. Thomas, 1965.

70. Neugarten, B. L. Patterns of aging: Past, present and future. *Social Service Review* 47: 571–580, 1973.

71. Odegaard, O. Emigration and insanity. *Acta Psychiatrica et Neurologica* 4: Supplement 4, 1932.

72. Park, B. *An Introduction to Telemedicine: Interactive Television for Delivery of Health Services.* New York: The Alternate Media Center, New York University, 1974.

73. Pearlin, L. I., & Schooler, C. The structure of coping. *Journal of Health and Social Behavior* 19: 2–21, 1978.

74. Perlin, M. L. *Rights of Ex-Patients in the Community: The Next Frontier.* Tape, Audio-Digest Psychiatry 9: 1, 1980. Audio-Digest Foundation, California.

75. Price, J. H., et al. The Lincolnshire Rehabilitation Scheme. *British Journal of Psychiatry* 115: 1043–1048, 1969.

76. Rabkin, J. G., & Struening, E. L. Life events, stress and illness. *Science* 194: 1013–1020, 1976.

77. Rahe, R. H., & Arthur, R. J. Life change and illness studies: Past history and future directions. *Journal of Human Stress* 4: 3–15, 1978.

78. Rahe, R. H. Life change events and mental illness: An overview. *Journal of Human Stress* 5:2–10, 1979.

79. Rahe, R. H., Tuffle, C. F., Suchor, R. J., & Arthur, R. J. Group therapy in outpatient management of post-MI patients. *Psychiatry in Medicine* 4: 77–88, 1973.

80. Raphael, B. Preventive intervention with the recently bereaved. *Archives of General Psychiatry* 34: 1450–1454, 1977.

81. Rogers, J., Vachon, M. L. S., Lyall, W. A. L., Sheldon, A., & Freeman, S. J. J. An urban widow-to-widow program: From demonstration model to independent community service. *Hospital and Community Psychiatry*, 1980.

82. Rogers, J., MacBride, A., Whylie, B., & Freeman, S. J. J. The use of groups in the rehabilitation of amputees. *International Journal of Psychiatry in Medicine* 8: (3), 243–255, 1977–78.

83. Rogers, M. P., Dubey, D., & Reich, P. The influence of the psyche and the brain on immunity and disease susceptibility: A critical review. *Psychosomatic Medicine* 41: (2), 147–164, 1979.

84. Rosen, B. M., Bahn, A. K., & Kramer, M. Demographic and diagnostic characteristics of psychiatric clinic outpatients in the U.S.A., 1961. *American Journal of Orthopsychiatry* 34: 455–468, 1964.

85. Roy, D. J., & Rausch, H. L. The psychiatric halfway house: How is it measuring up? *Community Mental Health Journal* 11: 155–162, 1975.

86. Schwenger, C. W. Health care for aging Canadians. *Canadian Welfare* 52: 9–12, 1977.

87. Schramm, C. J., & DeFillippi. Characteristics of successful alcoholism treatment programs for American workers. *British Journal of Addiction* 70: (3), 271–275, 1975.

88. Schwartz, M. D. Situation/transition groups: A conceptualization and review. *American Journal of Orthopsychiatry* 45: (5), 744–755, 1975.

89. Shonick, H. Premarital counseling: Three years experience of a unique service. *The Family Coordinator* 24: (3), 321–324, 1975.

90. Smith, H. C., & Hershenson, D. B. Attitude impact of vocational rehabilitation and psychotherapy on black poverty clients. *Journal of Applied Rehabilitation Counseling* 8: 33–38, 1977.

91. Sorensen, E. T. Group therapy in a community hospital dialysis unit. *Journal of the American Medical Association* 221: 899–901, 1972.

92. Stephenson, P. S., & Walker, G. A. The psychiatrist-woman patient relationship. *Canadian Journal of Psychiatry* 24: 5–17, 1979.

93. Straker, N., Mostyn, P., & Marshall, C. The use of two-way television in bringing mental health services to the inner city. *American Journal of Psychiatry* 133: 1202–1205, 1976.

94. Sunier, A. Mental illness and psychiatric care in Israel. In H. B. M. Murphy (ed.), *Social Changes and Mental Health. Milbank Memorial Fund Quarterly* 39: 385, 1956.

95. Talbott, J. A. Deinstitutionalization: Avoiding the disasters of the past. *Hospital and Community Psychiatry* 30: 621–624, 1979.

96. Vachon, M. L. S. Grief and bereavement following the death of a spouse. *Canadian Psychiatric Association Journal* 21: 35–43, 1976.

97. Vachon, M. L. S., Lyall, W. A. L., Rogers, J., Freedman, K., & Freeman, S. J. J. A controlled study of self-help intervention with windows. *American Journal of Psychiatry,* 1980.

98. Vachon, M. L. S., Lyall, W. A. L., Rogers, J., Formo, A., Freedman, K., Cochrane, J., Freeman, S. J. J. Use of group meetings with cancer patients and their families. In J. Tache, H. Selye, & S. B. Day (eds.), *Cancer, Stress and Death.* New York: Plenum Publishing Corp., 1979.

99. Walker, K., Rogers, J., & Messinger, L. Remarriage after divorce: A review. *Social Casework* 58: 276–285, 1977.

100. Warheit, G. J. Life events, coping, stress and depressive symptomatology. *American Journal of Psychiatry* 136: 502–507, 1979.

101. Wasylenki, D., & Freeman, S. J. J. Crises of living. In S. E. Greben, R. Pos, V. Rakoff, A. Bonkalo, F. H. Lowy, & G. Voineskos (eds.), *A Method of Psychiatry.* Philadelphia: Lea and Febiger, 1980.

102. Wasylenki, D. Depression in the elderly. *Canadian Medical Association Journal* 122: 525–533, 1980.

103. Weiss, R. S. Transition states and other stressful situations: Their nature

and programs for their management. In G. Caplan & M. Killilea (eds.), *Support Systems and Mutual Help: Multidisciplinary Explorations,* pp. 213–232. New York: Grune and Stratton, 1976.

104. Winnick, L., & Robbins, G. F. Physical and psychologic readjustment after mastectomy. *Cancer* 39: 478–486, 1977.

105. Winslow, W. W. The changing role of psychiatrists in community mental health centers. *American Journal of Psychiatry* 136: 24–27, 1979.

106. Zilbarth Junghardt, D. A program of postvention. In C. L. Hatton, S. M. Valente, & A. Rink (eds.), *Suicide: Assessment and Intervention.* New York: Appleton-Century-Crofts, 1977.

Psychiatry in Hungary, A Comparative View: Progress in the Hungarian Mental Health Care System, From Far behind Coming into the Limelight

John Furedi, M.D., Ph.D.

The subtitle of this paper may surprise you. You might wonder at the expression "far behind," because Hungary has given the world such names as Meduna, Ferenczi, Melanie Klein, Sandor Rado, Franz Alexander, Michael Balint, Thomas Szasz, and many others. Yet how could Hungary come into the limelight when hardly anybody knows about contemporary Hungarian psychiatry. However, these statements are illusive as all the famous people mentioned before were indeed born in Hungary, but sooner or later they left the country and were professionally successful in the West. On the other hand, those who know only a little of the present situation in Hungary will, I hope, get to know much more about it in the near future, as more and more Hungarian psychiatrists are participating in different international psychiatric associations all over the world. Thus, a good opportunity is given to impart knowledge about our endeavors, and I hope that psychiatrists visiting Europe will come in increasing numbers to Hungary to get personal impressions as well. Now, on this occasion I would like to give some details about the present-day situation.

The relative backwardness of Hungarian psychiatry has many causes. The first mental hospital was established only in 1850 and there were no more than two built since then. All other psychiatric wards have been established in general hospitals. However, these wards were poorly supplied and staffed because of the low priority that the general hospitals and the government set on psychiatric services. On the other hand we have at least avoided large mental hospitals. This effort becomes clear from Table 1 by comparing the number of beds in different settings in England, West Germany, and Hungary.

The other inhibiting factors were that for many years only the traditional German orientation was accepted. Although the Hungarian Psychoanalytic Association was one of the very first to be established, it never gained ground in official psychiatry. Partly because the association was seen by the fascists as a Jewish preoccupation and therefore it was persecuted. Later the association was judged to be an idealistic philosophy and neglected for this reason.

The situation did not become easier after World War II. Most hospitals were in ruins, and in the era of reconstruction, many other areas had priority over psychiatry, for example, tuberculosis, which was known as "Morbus Hungaricus." However, in the late sixties the situation changed. Dissatisfaction with custodial care had risen, and the attention of young psychiatrists had turned toward dynamic and social psychiatry. New methods of group therapy and rehabilitation

Table 1
Percentage of Beds in Different Psychiatric Units

Number of Beds	Hungary	West Germany	England
50	11.1 ⎫ 31.7	1.2	4.5
51— 100	20.6 ⎭		
101— 200	41.3 ⎫ 63.5	9.5	10.6
201— 500	22.2 ⎭		
501—1000	3.2	21.3	33.6
1001	1.6	68.0	51.3
TOTAL	100%	100%	100%

became more widespread in many parts of the country and the financial situation had changed to the better. The anti-tuberculosis program achieved many good results and thus made it possible to build new psychiatric wards or to transform the tuberculosis sanatoriums into psychiatric units. In 1966 a new regulation was published that made voluntary admission to a psychiatric facility possible. In 1969 a directive was issued in which the need for progress in mental health care was laid down. The result of this endeavor is shown in Tables 2 and 3. The number of beds has risen significantly, and the distribution of beds in the country has gradually become more even. Compared with other medical branches in Hungary, the psychiatric development has been one of the most dynamic. This development has been reflected in the increased number of discharges.

We had to admit, however, that the establishment of comprehensive, well-staffed outpatient services somehow was neglected, although there was no question about their growth in number (Table 4). It became evident that good results were not obtained where in- and outpatient services were strictly separated. Emphasis was laid mainly on expanding inpatient beds and personnel. Much higher respect was shown to psychiatrists working in an inpatient ward rather than those in an outpatient setting.

It was recognized that we needed a new system that would lead to a more efficient care of patients. The new ideology could be charac-

Table 2
Percentage of Inpatient Facilities for 10,000 Population

Ward	For 10,000 Population					
	1960	1965	1970	1972	1975	1976
Intern	10.5	11.6	13.8	14.2	14.7	15.5
Surgery	9.0	9.4	10.4	10.6	11.0	11.2
Child	6.9	7.4	8.1	8.1	8:1	8.3
Neurology	1.6	2.4	2.7	2.8	3.0	3.2
Psychiatry	6.8	7.2	7.8	8.3	9.9	10.1
TOTAL	69.6	75.8	80.9	82.1	84.2	86.0

Table 3
Percentage of Discharges For 1 Bed in Different Wards

Ward	1960	1965	1970	1975	1976
Intern	23.7	24.4	23.8	24.2	24.6
Surgery	26.8	27.1	27.0	26.2	26.3
Child	21.1	20.9	20.5	22.7	21.9
Neurology	14.8	14.8	15.8	17.2	17.0
Psychiatry	4.1	4.4	4.9	6.1	6.0
TOTAL	20.4	20.6	21.3	21.7	21.6

Table 4
Hours at Disposal for Outpatient Service in Hungary

Year	Hours
1955	119.5
1960	128.0
1965	233.0
1970	409.0
1975	684.0
1980	956.6

Number of Psychiatrists Working Fulltime
in Outpatient Services

1969	59
1980	160

terized by two words: *integration* and *progressiveness*. In our conception, integration means a comprehensive care system where all facilities are brought together in the framework of an integrated department. The department has one physician in charge who is responsible for prevention, out- and inpatient treatment, and rehabilitation of a certain population. Therapists and other health workers belonging to the same team can rotate in the system according to a particular plan.

However, it was understood that not all kinds of services can be organized in every hospital or every district. Thus child psychiatric departments could be available only in certain hospitals, but outpatient care is needed in every town. Different levels of rehabilitation, day and night hospitals, sheltered workshops, etc. are not necessarily sufficient in all settings but are efficient in the well-organized facilities. The cooperation between large and small institutions has been established according to this idea. This effort is called the *progressive* care system.

Integration and progressivity became the leading principles of the Hungarian medical care system. However, in its fulfillment there were many difficulties. The Ministry of Health and its regulation could give only the directives for the establishment of an advanced system, but its execution has at times been inhibited by narrow-mindedness or concern for loss of power. In the field of psychiatry experienced but old-fashioned professionals tried for many years to put obstacles in the way of integration. To overcome these difficulties it seemed practical to organize a model-department where we could try to work according to these ideas of integration. For this purpose our unit was established in the State Central Hospital in Budapest.

To start with there was no psychiatric service at that institution where I have been active for many years. The task of psychiatric care was partly put upon the neurology ward, or patients were transferred to other institutions in Budapest. According to Hungarian tradition some of the physicians working in neurological departments carried out psychiatric treatment as well. Although they did their best, the structure and possibilities of the neurological ward made it impossible to offer a full service. The separate jurisdictions of these two specialities had first to be established. We regarded it vitally important that psychotics, alcoholics, and patients with personality disturbances be treated in a psychiatric department. We understood that for idealogical reasons it was inevitable to exclude neurotics from any department of the hospital, but the most difficult cases were sent to our ward. Patients with psychotic episodes due to organic illnesses, vascular brain syndroms, and psychophysiological cases had to be determined on an individual basis as to where they were to be treated. Besides our organizational conception we had to take into consideration the physical conditions we had at our disposal. Accordingly we set up a special form of ward structure that first seemed to be too complicated. Nevertheless, it turned out to be the best solution to fulfill the needs of our patients.

Our institution is located near the center of Buda (the old part of Budapest) within a seven-story hospital, adjacent to which there is a four-story building where the outpatient consulting rooms are located. Under such circumstances our outpatient service is to be found among the other medical facilities having no difficulty in access in this setting. We have two well-separated and one partly separated rooms to ensure the privacy of individual or group psychotherapy. One floor houses the acute admissions. There we have four rooms with a total of 14 beds. The rooms have different sizes. Thus we are able to change the male and female wards, according to needs. Besides the ward rooms, we have three consulting rooms, one for minor surgery, one lounge, and one room for administration. Our institute has an establishment in the Buda hills in a distance of three kilometers from the mother institute. There we have on the same location two buildings: one for medical and one for psychiatric rehabilitation. This second one is a two-story building, very comfortable, fully equipped with only 14 beds. We decided not to have medical signs in this building. The staff wears no white coats here, and we have no surgery or other medical procedures. Since we have sufficient space in this setting we could organize a day treatment program from 8:30 A.M. until 3:30 P.M. Under such circumstances we can offer nearly a full service for our population. However, I am certain that in the near future we shall need some psychogeriatric facilities and at least an outpatient child service as well. Many experts may think that under such conditions we will not be able to fulfill our task, since our institute is responsible for a population of 38,000, which means that we have only 7.6 beds for 10,000 people. This ratio is much below the Hungarian average,

12.2 per 10,000 in 1980. In spite of some differing opinions, I strongly believe that if we continue to be well staffed and are able to establish a systematic working method and therapeutic milieu, we shall be able to survive well.

In terms of staffing, five of us are working in the integrated department as psychiatrists; further, two psychologists, one social worker, one occupational therapist, two administrators, and nineteen nurses complete the staff. Only the nurses have a regular working place. All the other members of the staff follow the patients to the different sections. It means that each patient has got the same therapist, physician, or psychologist, regardless of his/her inpatient or aftercare status. With this integrated service we can keep the contact continuously with all patients outside the hospital, whenever needed, so that there is no need to keep them too long in the hospital.

In the first year, when only half as many beds were available we had treated 205 patients, but in the second year we treated 450 and in the third, 483 cases. The distribution of our patients in the different sections and their average length of stay is shown in Table 5. It becomes clear from the table that some patients after a partial recovery were transferred from the acute unit to the rehabilitation section. However, some patients got treatment primarily in one of the services only. According to our principles, the acute unit is led mainly in the medical, short-term, diagnostic, or emergency model. On the other hand the rehabilitation unit, in- and outpatient wards, work along the idea of a therapeutic community. There, individual and group psychotherapy, large and small, psychodrama, and other kinds of group activities (music therapy, exercising, etc.) are the main therapeutic methods.

This interchangeable option resulted in a short stay in both inpatient sections. To compare with the Hungarian average stay of 57.1 days, our organization had dramatically shortened the inpatient days. This progress would not have been possible if we had not emphasized the importance of outpatient services. For half a year one psychiatrist is working full time in the outpatient section and is responsible for this part of our service. The other psychiatrists work here once a week for a half day to interview their discharged patients or to accept any new urgent cases. Besides, there are follow-up groups to which the patients belong for a long time after their active treatment period. They

Table 5
Percentage of Length of Stay in the Two Inpatient Units

	No. of Cases	Inpatient Days	Average Length of Stay
Treated only in the admission unit	185	3411	18.4
Treated only in the rehabilitation unit	119	2134	17.9
Treated in both units	146		
Admission unit		2166	14.8
Rehabilitation unit		2665	18.2
		4831	33.1
All patients treated in the admission unit	331	5877	17.7
All patients treated in the rehabilitation unit	265	4799	18.1
TOTAL	450	10376	23.06

Table 6
Previous Occurrences Psychiatric Inpatient Treatment

Never been treated in any psychiatric inpatient ward	236 admissions
Treated, but not in our department	59 admissions
Treated only by us	33 admissions
Treated elsewhere and here too	34 admissions
Several treatments in other wards in the same year	88 admissions
TOTAL	450 admissions

Table 7

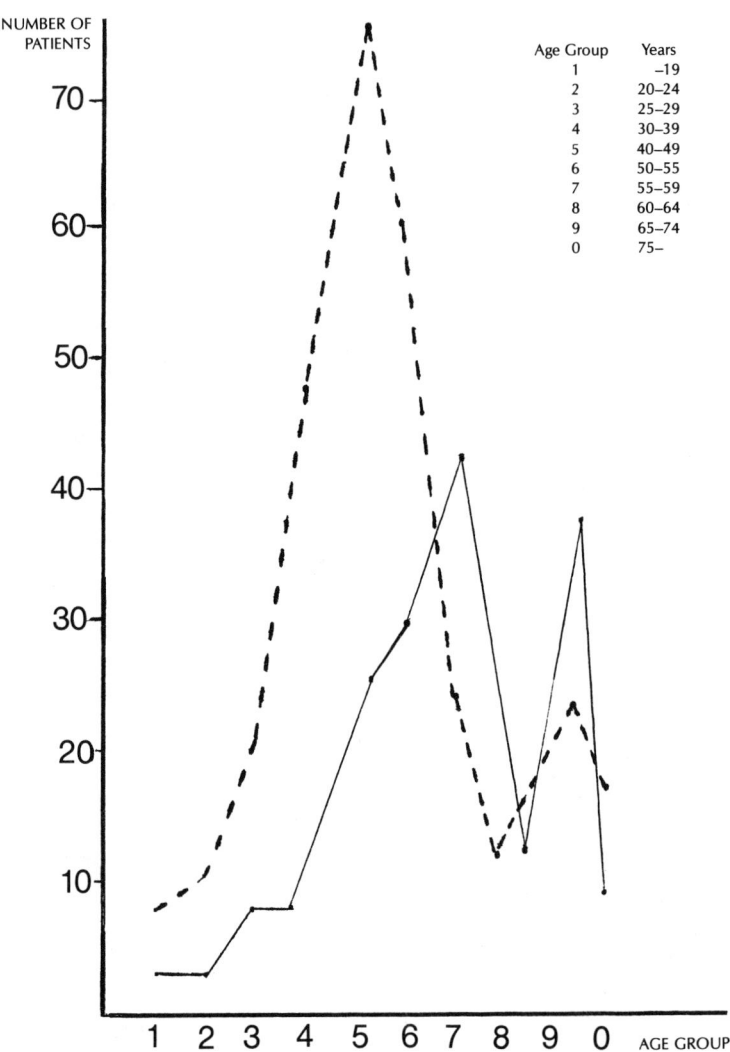

attend these groups after they have already returned home and to their original jobs. At present we have three groups running for more than two years and the psychodrama group has met for one year. In 1980 we had more than 12,000 patient visits.

In regard to our inpatients, the distribution by previous stay in a psychiatric inpatient facility, diagnosis, and length of stay, age, and sex is shown in Tables 6 and 7. Table 6 shows that half the patients in that ward were new admissions. This large number makes our task more interesting but harder at the same time. We have more female than male patients primarily in the middle age range. The diagnoses cover the full psychiatric nomenclature as a reflection of the comprehensive service our department offers.

We hope that the model we have evolved will stimulate the future establishment of further progressive and integrated mental health facilities in Hungary.

Present Status and the Future of Outpatient Drug Management of Schizophrenia

Yvon D. Lapierre, M.D.

The discovery of chlorpromazine in 1952 (4) and its application to mental illness revolutionized the treatment approaches to schizophrenia. Patients who previously have been condemned to a lifetime in psychiatric institutions were now able to benefit more effectively from the psychosocial approaches that were coming forth at that time. Thus, they could lead lives that were closer to normality. Within a very short time span, psychiatric institutions saw their resident population decrease by leaps and bounds and psychiatric patients started migrating either to their community of origin or to alternate accommodations more in keeping with normal society. Although many of these patients were readmitted to hospital, inpatient stays remained briefer and social functioning was maintained in cases where such a possibility would have been unheard of prior to 1952.

These schizophrenic patients were not cured by any means. Nevertheless, the secondary symptoms of the illness that affect intrapsychic and social behavior were sufficiently controlled to allow for hospital discharge. These symptoms, generally referred to as the positive symptoms of schizophrenia, include hallucinations, delusions, agitation, all of which usually come under the control of neuroleptics. The alleviation of these symptoms all contributed to facilitating the return to the community. The so-called negative symptoms, on the other hand, such as autism, apathy, and loss of drive did not respond as well to these pharmacotherapeutic agents. This differential effectiveness led to an increased number of patients discharged from hospital but the persistence of the remaining core symptoms resulted in increasing demands for rehabilitation. Whereas, previously, social problems associated with mental illness were hidden away in the back wards of large institutions, this efflux of patients necessitated increased social awareness and manpower to cope with the large number of patients requiring aftercare.

Costs that were limited previously to resident custodial care rose with more active therapeutic intervention leading to increased demands on the taxpayers. This financial burden inevitably led to a reassessment of treatment effectiveness. The initial therapeutic expectations from psychotropic agents were probably unrealistic, but the scientific methods of assessment introduced early in this era allowed for objective verification and objectification of pharmacotherapy. This outcome was not necessarily the case for other forms of treatment.

The efficacy of neuroleptics has been studied from different perspectives (3, 5). Placebo-controlled studies of neuroleptics in acute psychosis demonstrated the superiority of the active drug in the acute phase of the illness. Once the acute phase has subsided, however, the therapeutic results are less striking and their objective assessment is also more difficult. As mentioned earlier, neuroleptics are not as effective against the so-called negative symptoms of schizophrenia as they are against the psychotic elaborations. Therefore, assessment of drug efficacy must consider other variables of change in addition to obvious psychopathology. These criteria of therapeutic efficacy have included relapse rates, rehospitalization rates, direct costs, etc.

The studies of Hogarthy (7) demonstrated the superiority of chlorpromazine over a placebo in preventing relapse and rehospitalization. These same studies also brought out the importance of major role therapy in the follow-up care of these patients. The synergism of combined psychotherapeutic and pharmacotherapeutic approaches on the reduction of relapses and subsequent rehospitalizations persisted for the three years of the study.

On the basis of cost-benefits, neuroleptics may be considered as a relatively inexpensive method of treatment for schizophrenia (12). However, lower cost of active treatment alone should not lead one to hasty conclusions. The indirect costs of relapse into psychosis far exceed the direct costs of treatment. Loss of employment and economic stability, the impact on family life and thus on the eventual possibilities of rehabilitation are as difficult to assess in financial terms as is quality of life. A relapse leads to increased morbidity and can also lead to depression and suicide. In addition, there is evidence suggesting that relapses result in greater deterioration of the personality and thus to a more malignant course of the illness.

The discovery of neuroleptic drugs, as is often the case in medicine, came about somewhat fortuitously via another discipline, anaesthesiology. Although the understanding of their mechanisms of action on cerebral function lagged behind the demonstration of their usefulness, they have had definite heuristic value in research and on working hypotheses of schizophrenia. A major contribution they have had is in the conceptualization of schizophrenia as an illness. Although this disease concept of schizophrenia is still debated in many quarters, it is a useful way of approaching the condition and has contributed immensely to etiological research (6).

The neuropharmacological mechanism common to all neuroleptic drugs is their ability to block dopamine receptors in the brain. This action led to the elaboration of the dopamine hypothesis of schizophrenia, which in turn led to numerous studies that furthered the understanding of neuropharmacological mechanisms in vitro, in animals, and on human brain function. There is presently sufficient evidence to suggest that dopamine function is probably abnormal in schizophrenics. Whether this abnormality lies in the presynaptic neuron, in the synapse, or in the postsynaptic neuron is not yet clear. Nor is it altogether clear whether or not this dopamine abnormality is the etiological factor of the condition or an epiphenomenon of another as yet undiscovered abnormality. Nevertheless, knowledge resulting from neuroleptic research has served as an avenue of investigative research and further clarification of possible biological bases of this illness. This dopamine abnormality most probably involves the mesolimbic tract. As this pharmacological action of dopamine receptor blocking is not specific to this tract, the same effect in other parts of the brain contributes to many of the unwanted side effects of these drugs.

Blockage of dopamine receptors of the nigrostriatal tract is the cause of the extrapyramidal side effects often caused by neuroleptics. Blockage of the tubero-infundibular pathway results in the disinhibiting release of prolactin with resulting galactorrhea and menstrual irregularities. Dopamine blockage of the incerto-hypothalamic tract may result in the observed changes in temperature regulation. There are most probably other mechanisms that come into play which still remain undiscovered.

There are at least eight classes of drugs with demonstrated neuroleptic activity. Not all of these are available in the North American market (Table 1).

Chlorpromazine, a phenothiazine, was the first neuroleptic drug used clinically. Subsequently, other phenothiazines were synthesized, mainly through side-chain substitutions ending up with three biochemical groups now referred to as aliphatic, piperidine, and piperazine. These structural differences also account for different profiles of clinical activity. The aliphatic and piperidine compounds are also referred to as the high weight phenothiazines and the piperazine as the low weight. This measure reflects the amount of

Table 1
Drugs with Demonstrated Neuroleptic Activity

I. PHENOTHIAZINES
   A—Aliphatic:
      chlorpromazine
   B—Piperidine:
      thioridazine
      mezoridazine
   C—Piperazine:
      trifluoperazine
      perphenazine
      thioproperazine
II. BUTYROPHENONES
      haloperidol
      droperidol
III. DIPHENYLBUTYLPIPERIDINES
      pimozide
      fluspirilene
      penfluridol

IV. THIOXANTHENES
      thiothixene
      prochlorthixene
V. DIBENZOXAPINE
      loxapine
VI. DIBENZODIAZEPINE
      clozapine
VII. BENZAMIDES
      sulpiride
      sultopride
      tiapride
VIII. INDOLES
      molindone

drug, on a weight basis, that is required to achieve similar results. The occurrence of autonomic side effects is also more common with the aliphatic compounds than with the piperazine derivatives. On the other hand, extrapyramidal side effects are more common and more pronounced with the piperazine derivatives. Although sedation is more pronounced with the aliphatic group, the onset of antipsychotic activity is more rapid with the piperazine derivatives. The piperidine series generally has a profile closer to the aliphatics as far as side effects and clinical activity is concerned. On the other hand, the incidence of electrocardiographic changes is greater for these (9), and at high doses, thioridazine has been more associated with retinal changes than the other phenothiazines.

The butyrophenones represented a major departure from the phenothiazines and other psychotropics of the day as far as chemical structure is concerned. Only haloperidol is available in North America. It has a clinical therapeutic profile similar to the piperazine phenothiazines but has the added benefit of being less sedative. On the other hand, its use is associated with a high incidence of extrapyramidal side effects.

The molecular structure of the diphenylbutylpiperidines is similar to that of the butyrophenones. However, the clincial profile of this series is slightly different. The main difference observed with the diphenylbutylpiperidines is their effect on the negative symptoms of schizophrenia and the longer duration of action of fluspirilene and penfluridol.

Pimozide, administered once daily, has been demonstrated as improving the social interactions of chronic schizophrenics in group therapy (10). Penfluridol, a once weekly administered oral neuroleptic, produces less anergia over many months of administration than does fluphenazine (11).

A similar clinical response was also observed with long-term therapy with fluspirilene (Lapierre et al; in preparation). This group of drugs has more specific dopamine receptor blocking activity. They may be the drugs of choice in the treatment of the withdrawn apathetic schizophrenics.

The thioxanthenes have been in use for a number of years. Although their use is not as widespread as that of most other neuroleptics, they are often recommended for schizophrenics with depressive tendencies. Their overall profile of action is otherwise quite similar to the phenothiazines of the piperazine series (1).

The only dibenzoxapine available for clinical use is loxapine. It is an effective neuroleptic quite similar to the phenothiazines.

The dibenzodiazepine, clozapine, was a novel and important addition to the pharmacotherapeutic armamentarium against schizophrenia. For the first time, a neuroleptic drug was practically devoid of extrapyramidal activity. Although this drug was subsequently withdrawn from use because of its toxicity to the blood-forming organs, it did focus the attention of psychopharmacologists on a specific dopamine blocker of the mesolimbic tract and thus opened the door to further clarifications on the underlying illness. It is to be expected that a similar compound to clozapine with fewer of its toxic side effects will be developed (2).

More recently, two additional series of drugs have been introduced in the treatment of schizophrenia. The benzamides include three drugs having neuroleptic potential. Sulpiride, Sultopride, and Tiapride are presently under investigation in Europe (13). It is yet too early to compare their efficacy with the presently available neuroleptics.

Molindone, an indole compound, has a slightly different biochemical profile but is also in the early stages of comparison with the other neuroleptics (8).

Long-acting injectable neuroleptics were developed to overcome two major problems associated with chronic neuroleptic therapy. One of these is compliance. Any patient suffering from a chronic illness requiring daily drug intake is, by virtue of human failings, bound to be delinquent in his self-administration of medication. This normal reaction is compounded when cessation of the drug intake is associated with a brief feeling of improvement because of removal of its sedative effect plus the usual lack of immediate appreciable benefit from the drug. These factors, added on to frequent lack of insight or awareness of being ill, increase the risk of lack of compliance in the treatment of these patients.

The second major reason for developing long-acting injectables is to decrease the absolute amount of drug intake. This procedure may not prevent all of the side effects of long-term drug administration but certainly decreases the risks related to cumulation of drug in body stores.

Two types of long-acting injectable neuroleptics are presently available for the treatment of schizophrenia. These are the oily depot and the crystalline depot long-actings. The original preparations of depot neuroleptics was based on a well-recognized pharmaceutical method of combining the active ingredient with an organic acid to form an ester. The compounded drug is then injected in an oily vehicle that will cause it to be released still more slowly and to form secondary deposits in tissues of affinity. Representative drugs of most classes of neuroleptics have thus been prepared for depot administration (Table 2). These include piperidine and piperazine phenothiazines, thioxanthenes, and butyrophenones. The enanthate compounds have an average two weeks duration of effect whereas the decanoate and palmitate compounds have a duration of therapeutic action that varies from three to five or even six weeks.

The crystalline depot long-acting neuroleptic in use is Fluspirilene, a diphenylbutylpiperidine. It is generally administered once weekly.

The indications for continuing neuroleptic therapy and the preferential use of one compound over another are not easily defined for an individual patient. A combination of variables contributes to the decision of continuing neuroleptic therapy. The most important is the occurrence of relapse when neuroleptics are withdrawn. The persistence of symptoms even in a subacute form is an indication for continued medication.

Table 2
Long-Acting Neuroleptic Injectables

1 Week   ± : Fluspirilene
2 Weeks ± : Fluphenazine Enanthate
4 Weeks ± : Fluphenazine Decanoate
                Pipothiazine Palmitate
                Haloperidol Decanoate
                Flupenthixol Decanoate

Well-defined target symptoms and individual patient characteristics then serve as guides to the choice of drug.

The objectives of drug therapy in chronic schizophrenics are: (1) return to function, (2) maintenance of function, (3) a decrease and cessation of symptoms, and (4) minimization of side effects. These objectives are to be kept in mind when deciding on initiation of drug therapy and whether to change or continue a preestablished treatment program.

The decision of long-term use of long-acting injectables is sometimes a difficult one. Oral administration has many psychological advantages. The patient remains in control of his/her medication and any threat to his/her self-determination and individuality is at a minimum. However, this control must be balanced with the possibility of diminished compliance and cumulative side effects. Injectables have been demonstrated as of superior effectiveness in reducing the incidence of relapse. The effectiveness of injectable neuroleptics is generally three times that of oral administration in controlling symptoms and has been associated with a sevenfold decrease in relapse rate. The use of injectables overcomes problems of absorption, and compliance ensures continued contact with the treatment team. Best results are obtained generally with injectables when the decision to use them is a joint patient-therapist process.

Future developments in the drug therapy of schizophrenia can be expected in two general areas: the first will be related to refinements in the use of presently available medication, and the second will be in exploration of new frontiers.

The criteria for drug administration will become better defined. The decision on indications for drug administration will be further clarified to include differences due to sex, race, and genetic loading. The prediction of drug responsiveness using biological markers such as neurohormones will be more clearly defined.

Monitoring of blood levels will remain a problem for some time because of the great number of active metabolites of these drugs. However, functional blood levels of neuroleptics will be more easily and more cheaply determined using tests such as the presently developing radio-receptor assays.

New drugs will be developed. Clozapine-like compounds with more specific actions at better defined brain sites will permit further insights into brain function in normality and in illness. With developments of specificity of drug site of action will also follow more precise diagnoses of schizophrenia and clarification of subgroups in this heterogenous group of illnesses.

To decrease the risk of side effects to neuroleptic administration, non-neuroleptic drugs will be added to the former to potentiate their therapeutic actions while using lower doses. One route through which this goal may be achieved is with GABA-like drugs. Long-acting neuroleptics will be developed along the lines of penfluridol. This type of drug, administered orally once weekly, is a more ideal long-acting neuroleptic than are the depot injectables.

Associated with these drug developments, neuropharmacological substrates of schizophrenia will continue to be researched, the dopamine hypothesis will certainly be modified, and as mechanisms of secondary messenger systems in the postsynaptic neurons become more clearly defined, specific defects in schizophrenic brain function will become clearer.

Other neurotransmitters are yet to be discovered and explored further. In spite of the voluminous literature emanating from neurosciences, very little is really known about brain mechanisms. One day thought processes may also be understood on a biochemical basis thus permitting more specific remedies for this malignant illness.

References

1. Ban, T. A. *Psychopharmacology of Thiothixene*. New York: Raven Press Books, 1978.

2. Beckman, B., Hippius, H., & Ruther, E. Treatment of schizophrenia. *Progress in Neuropsychopharmacology* 3: 47–52, 1979.

3. Davis, J. M. Recent developments in the drug treatment of schizophrenia. *American Journal of Psychiatry* 133: (2), 208–214, February 1976.

4. Delay, J., & Deniker, P. 38 cas de psychose traités par la cure prolongée et continue de 4568 RP. *Annals of Medical Psychology* 110: (36), 4, 1952.

5. Gardos, G., & Cole, J. O. Maintenance antipsychotic therapy: Is the cure worse than the disease? *American Journal of Psychiatry* 133: (1), 32–36, January 1976.

6. Hemmings, G. Concept of disease in psychiatry. *Journal of the Royal Society of Medicine* 73: 154, February 1980.

7. Hogarty, G. E., & Goldberg, S. C. Collaborative study group: Drug and sociotherapy in the aftercare of schizophrenic patients: One-year relapse rates. *Archives of General Psychiatry* 28: 54–64, 1973.

8. Kellner, R., Rada, R. T., Egelman, A., & Macaluso, G. Long-term study of molindone hydrochloride in chronic schizophrenics. *Current Therapeutic Research* 20, 5 November 1976.

9. Lapierre, Y. D., Lapointe, L., Bordeleau, J. M., & Tetreault, L. Phenothiazine treatment and electrocardiographic abnormalities—A survey of 106 psychiatric patients receiving thioridazine. *Canadian Psychiatric Association Journal* 14: 517–523, 1968.

10. Lapierre, Y. D. Pimozide and the social behavior of schizophrenics. *Current Therapeutic Research*. 18: (1), Section 2, 181–188, July 1975.

11. Lapierre, Y. D. A controlled study of penfluridol in the treatment of schizophrenics. *American Journal of Psychiatry* 135: (8), 956–959, August 1978.

12. May, P. R. A. Cost efficiency of treatments for the schizophrenic patient. *American Journal of Psychiatry* 127: (10), 382–385, April 1971.

13. Ropert, R., Caillard, F., & Petitjean, F. Benzamides and related compounds. *University of Ottawa Psychiatric Journal* 4: (2), 161–169, June 1979.

Sex Therapy in the 1980s

Domeena C. Renshaw, M.B., Ch.B., M.D.

It is worthwhile, at the start of a new decade, to review what has been accomplished in the preceding one in the field of sex therapy. While sexual dysfunctions are probably as old as the human race, it is only within the last ten years that highly successful brief outpatient treatment techniques have been discovered and duplicated. It is barely fourteen years ago that the basic mechanisms of male and female sexual responses were definitively and scientifically studied and documented in St. Louis, Missouri, by William Masters, M.D., a gynecologist (3, 4).

Causes and cures for sexual dysfunctions have preoccupied both physicians and charlatans for centuries (2). Theories of etiologies have varied from punishment (either divine or diabolical) to established organic pathology (2, 8). Yet, despite the long and well-documented list of possible pathology, organic causes of permanent sexual dysfunctions are less common than emotional etiology. Transient episodes of sexual problems with minimal organicity but much emotional overlay have been known to lead to unnecessary persistence of symptomatology long after adequate medical treatment of the acute condition, such as prostatitis, vaginitis, drug or alcohol side-effects, etc.

What are sexual dysfunctions? A simple definition is exceptionally difficult to formulate. The following definition has been useful:

Sexual dysfunctions are impaired, incomplete, or absent expressions of normally recurrent human sexual desires and responses. Difficulties with pleasurable sexual arousal or climactic resolution then occur. Sexual functioning becomes problematic or symptomatic only when there is subjective discomfort related to a dysfunction. Partner dissatisfaction, however, may for the first time precipitate awareness of a dysfunction as occurs in premature ejaculation in a man who, himself, attains release yet wishes to please his partner by a sustained erection.

Sexual expression has wide variations, is governed by personal values/inhibitions, and is culturally determined upon innate individual drives. Mutuality is attained with effort, experience, compromise, commitment, maturity, and considerate interpersonal exchange. There is a wide difference between making sex and making love. Fortunate couples may attain the closeness and the intimacy to do both.

In the past, treatment of sexual dysfunctions has been singularly unsuccessful. Years of psychoanalysis and individual psychotherapy may have provided knowledge of *why* the symptom developed, but afforded minimal relief (14). The critical gap was the shroud of mystery around the coital act, and scientific ignorance regarding the drama of sexual climax. The universal phenomenon of orgasm was not easily taught or described until this decade. The old response to an inquiring female patient, "If you've had one, you'd know one," from gynecologists is no longer defensible. Direct explicit questions like: "What happens to your breathing/heart rate/muscles/vaginal secretions? Do you feel some contractions in your arms, legs, and vagina?" All of these questions may be sexually educative. Also directed self-help reading may be of value (11).

For the average male, orgasm is confirmed by ejaculation. For the average female, it was cloaked in misinformation, myth, fantasy, and fog (1, 11). This outcome is now unnecessary. At any age, from in utero to the senium, a definition of orgasm is: a build-up of vasoneuromuscular genital tensions that culminate in a peak, with a sudden discharge of tensions, followed by a return to the preexcitement state (16). During sexual arousal, there is an increase in heart rate, respiratory rate, blood pressure and muscle tone, penile erection, and vaginal lubrication (3). From earliest childhood, the stimulus may be self (masturbation or fantasy), another person (same or opposite sex), or another species (animal) (5). All persons may be born with similar genital apparatus, but capacities to be aroused and to respond differ. This latter capacity depends on intact brain, spinal cord, peripheral and autonomic nerves plus muscles, blood vessels, and end organs; it also depends on external erotic stimuli (pleasurable, painful) plus socially learned inhibitions (6, 16).

Sexual expression is the only instinct where deliberate, sustained control or even complete suppression does not result in a threat to the life of the individual, as would cutting off breathing, eating, elimination, or circulation. This fact must be considered in cases where "loss of desire" is the presenting complaint. There may be intentional avoidance and possibly a *selective* nonfunction with this partner, while regular masturbation (or extra-marital sex) continues. In other cases loss of libido may be part of a clinical depression needing antidepressants (7) or even an anxious aversion to sex of phobic proportions requiring understanding, sex education, and directed desensitization.

Since 1970, thousands of "sex clinics" have appeared with no quality control or licensure requirements for those who call themselves "sex therapists." Physicians are concerned that in this highly sensitive area, vulnerable patients must be advised to check credentials carefully to prevent exploitation. Reputable sex clinics recognize the great amount of time that needs to be given to training sex therapists, whether this be the Masters-Johnson Institute at St. Louis or modifications of their described techniques (9, 15). Each would-be sex therapist brings his or her own sexual anxieties and attitudes into training and treatment (12). For all of us, sex is an area of human functioning that is highly sensitive, and heavily loaded with stored earlier memories of both pleasant and painful previous sexual stimuli, either real or fantasized. Also sexual expression is inextricably bound with personal values (12). This fact is as true for each therapist as it is for each patient. We need an understanding and acceptance of our own sexuality to enhance our therapeutic effectiveness. The more comfortable the physician, the more comfortable the patient. Also critical is that we not use our own sexual function/desire/history as an ideal index for the patients. It is *their* optimum sexual capacity we must understand and accept as the framework within which they will be able to function.

An exceptional standard of excellence and professionalism is demanded of those who would make ongoing contributions into sexual medicine. Those who seek sexual solutions or gratification for self in this intensely intimate and demanding modality can only bring discredit to their discipline and disaster to self and their vulnerable patients. A supervised training experience for the therapist allows for open discussion of these feelings in supervision (9, 15). This training enhances growth and prevents intrusion of the therapist's own sexual hang-ups into the patient's therapy. The use of two therapists, although expensive, assists by allowing continuing "in process" on site feedback, as they discuss the therapy in supervision breaks during actual clinical sessions. Much candor, intimacy, and exchange are demanded in sex therapy. Solo clinicians are also effective with solo patients or with couples.

Directive behavior modification techniques together with conjoint psychotherapy forms the main methodological underpinning of what is being called "The New Sex Therapy" (2). It is a breakthrough in the treatment of sexual dysfunctions, even those of twenty to thirty years duration; this brief behaviorally oriented outpatient sex therapy is effective from as short as two weeks (Masters-Johnson model) to modifications taking seven weeks (4, 9). Masters and Johnson have been criticized for being "simplistic," "mechanical," "cookbook," but their described techniques *do* work (4). The immediate results are highly effective, but the difficult task of follow-up is essential for careful ongoing scientific evaluation as to whether the improvements are sustained.

The basic principles of the Masters and Johnson sex therapy are those of competent medical practice: first, an extensive, explicit medical, sexual, and life history from each partner of a committed couple, and second, a careful physical examination from top to toe for each, and finally, sex education by the physician. Some important innovations they introduced were:

1. A dual-sex therapist team, so each patient partner is adequately represented and understood.

2. Specific "sexological examination" of each partner, symptomatic or not, by the responsible team M.D. in the presence of the spouse plus both members of the dual-sex therapy team. This personal education, in full light with a mirror for patient self-viewing, removes the cloak of mystery, myth, and misinformation around the genitals. The therapists clarify, encourage later questioning, and promote acceptance of the sight and feel of the sexual apparatus as natural, respectable, and potentially pleasurable in the privacy of their home.

3. Explaining comfortably and explicitly to the couple the anatomy and physiology of male and female sexual organs in all the phases of sexual responses, using some basic visual aids. Also, allowing the

couple to discuss any mistaken beliefs that may be causing them shame, anxiety, or guilt.

4. Suggesting for home practice behavioral changes for the couple to practice in the privacy of their own bedroom (new learning). The goal is to break old maladaptive, unsatisfactory sexual patterns, and replace them with different, less upsetting (pain avoidance), relaxing sensate body massage (reciprocal inhibition) and more enjoyable (positive pleasure/reward) responses. The natural reinforcements are most effective: enjoyable personal body reactions and positive verbal responses from partner and from therapists.

However, there may be many layers of interpersonal problems and conflicts between the couple, above and beyond the sexual problems. Which of these (marital conflict or sexual discordance) is primary and which is secondary may be merely academic by the time they reach sex therapy. Therefore, relationship or conjoint therapy must be combined with the sexual exercises. It is very interesting that the "New Sex Therapy" has so rapidly attained popular acceptability. Many call the Loyola Psychiatric Department requesting sex therapy, always insisting that they do not have psychiatric problems and do not need the psychiatric clinic, but readily attend the "sex clinic" (which uses the same outpatient space, billing, etc.)

A great deal more than "simple behavior therapy" occurs in the intense intimate exchange of sex therapy. Trust in the therapists as credible, concerned authorities is essential. Reassurance, direction, and permission to change sexual behavior is given to each. Destructive partner exchange is interpreted to the couple, often repeatedly, when there is resistance to resolving maladaptive relationship discord. Inevitably, couple psychotherapy is done. Which psychotherapy technique applied depends upon the therapists, as may the labeling of that technique (be this "none" as some sex therapists need to insist, marriage counseling, transactional analysis, or psychodynamic). All of these techniques have in common the inclusion of a sexual behavior focus, a time-limited contract, and explicit inquiry about their progress each visit to understand conflictual "blocking" of pleasurable sexual exchange. One-to-one therapy is avoided since the focus of treatment is the relationship of the couple. In effect one goal is partner-transference rather than therapist-transference.

At the risk of oversimplification, some common etiological factors must be considered in all sexual dysfunctions:

1. Anxiety about impregnation, venereal disease, pain, aging/looks, sinfulness, possible stroke, sexual performance, being discovered, or other priorities such as finances, domestic problems, need for sleep, etc.

2. Anger at oneself or each other, old remembered conflicts or current ones, resentments, etc.

3. The use of alcohol in excess. This problem is perhaps the commonest world-wide cause of the *first* episode of secondary impotence in males (13). When interpreted with high anxiety and fear of future performance, psychogenic impotence may become fixed.

4. Clinical depression, with its lowering of all appetites, whether for food, sleep, sex, and life (7).

5. Drugs, even lifesaving medications, may interfere with sexual performance (13).

6. One partner deliberately controlling the sexual exchange. This manipulation may be a unilateral decision in a relationship where there was a previous contract to share sexual expression. Conflict may surface when this event unfolds.

7. A dissociation of sexual feelings, i.e., an unconscious unwillingness to accept the sexual aspect of self, literally treating the sex organs as a nonpart of self, with massive denial (even aversion) of sexual sensations.

A trained therapist must also know the variety of ways in which different persons, cultures, religions, and age groups usually express and control their sexuality to avoid misinterpretation of a particular couple's history (6). For each culturally bound individual sex education (for better or for worse) results in sanctions or prohibitions that may be retained for life or that may be altered as they grow and learn sexual alternatives. A couples' interpersonal expression during a sexual exchange is always the ultimate outcome of the attitudes and ambivalences of the total person: toward beauty/ugliness, joy/guilt, pleasure/pain. Antecedent factors responsible for shaping sexual attitudes usually emerge during sex therapy. Without such personal background history for each patient, the therapist cannot bring into the couples' understanding of their sexual complaint lasting therapeutic perspective to assist with symptom-removal plus resultant general improvement in the relationship.

Finally, it bears reflection that differentiating between functional and physical sexual dysfunctions (for males) is finally possible today thanks to the modern technology called nocturnal penile plethysmography, which measures nocturnal penile tumescence (NPT) (8). For many conditions such as stroke, open heart surgery, renal dialysis, diabetes, hypertension (although medications may be causative), sexual dysfunction may be tragically fixed when the patient asks a sexual question and the physician prematurely states (without objective testing) that the sex problem is due to the disease. Most often this problem is found in a male who presents with impotence. He should first be sent for NPT tests to a urology department in a university to establish whether in the unconscious, uninhibited state of sleep there are good erections, indicating good penile function. Then the impotence is not due to organic or chemical factors. Sex clinics today merit a diagnostic trial for such patients also when there is ambiguity with noted emotional overlay upon some organic illness. Moreover, sex therapy has repeatedly proved of therapeutic value. One self-referred case of a diabetic male (who was relieved in week two of secondary impotence at Loyola) volunteered "my doctor told me not to waste your time and my money to go to a Sex Clinic" (10).

It is important that we, as physicians, retain sensitivity to the complaints of our patients including today their highly treatable sex problems. With all persons, including those with chronic problems of arthritis, alcoholism, diabetes, stroke, cardiac, renal, respiratory or skin diseases and with spinal injury, a sexual history should be a routine part of their medical history. This history takes a little extra time on the part of the physician but it is necessary to understand in depth and detail the many myths and misinformations gathered by the patient.

A great deal can be done by simple sex education from a respected physician authority. Many alternatives of sexual pleasuring can be suggested to promote the closeness, caring, and sharing needed especially in the stress of chronic illness. There is a difference between making sex (mechanical intercourse only) and making love (emotional nurturance). As stated earlier, some couples share both. We can teach them the difference so they may grow and choose. It is perhaps redundant to emphasize that, as holistic and humanistic physicians, we also strive to improve the quality of the lives we try to save.

References

1. Heiman, LoPiccolo, & LoPiccolo. *Becoming Orgasmic*. Englewood Cliffs, N.J.: Prentice-Hall, 1978.

2. Holbrook, S. *The Golden Age of Quackery*. New York: Macmillan, 1959.

3. Masters, William H., & Johnson, Virginia E. *Human Sexual Response*. Boston: Little, Brown, 1970.

4. Masters, William H., & Johnson, Virginia E. *Human Sexual Inadequacy*. Boston: Little, Brown, 1970.

5. Renshaw, Domeena C. Sexuality in children. *Medical Aspects of Human Sexuality* 5: X, pp. 65–74, October 1971.

6. Renshaw, Domeena C. Sex education for educators. *Journal of School Health* XLIII: 10, December 1973.

7. Renshaw, Domeena C. Sexual dysfunction in depression. *Psychosomatic Manifestations of Depression*, Ari Kiev, Editor, *Excerpta Medica*, Amsterdam, pp. 86–105, 1974.

8. Renshaw, Domeena C. Impotence—some causes and cures. *American Family Physician* 17: 2, pp. 143–146, February 1978.

9. Renshaw, Domeena C. Physician sexuality training program—a unique elective. *Chicago Medicine* 77: 21, pp. 868–870, October 19, 1974.

10. Renshaw, Domeena C. Impotence in diabetes. *Journal of Nervous and Mental Disorders* 36, pp. 369–371, July 1975.

11. Renshaw, Domeena C. Sex and the female psyche. *Comprehensive Therapy* 4: 5, pp. 17–21, May 1978.

12. Renshaw, Domeena C. Sex and values. *Journal of Clinical Psychiatry* 39, pp. 716–719, 1978.

13. Renshaw, Domeena C. Sex and drugs. *South African Medical Journal* 54, pp. 322–326, 1978.

14. Sherfey, M. J. The evolution and nature of female sexuality in psychoanalytic theory. *Journal of American Psychoanalytic Association* 14, pp. 28–128, 1966.

15. Waggoner, R. W., et al. Training dual-sex teams for rapid treatment of sexual dysfunction: a pilot program. *Psychiatric Annals* III: 5, pp. 61–76, May 1973.

16. Weiss, H. D. The physiology of human penile erections. *Annals of Internal Medicine* 76, pp. 793–799, 1972.

Bones of Contention in Group Psychotherapy

John T. Salvendy, M.D.

From the very beginning the theory and practice of group psychotherapy were accompanied by tones of dissent. Even its earliest infancy has been marred by the scandalous start Moreno gave in 1911 after he had started his first therapy group consisting of young Viennese prostitutes. Most of the first group therapists were psychoanalysts. The influence of this group is still a major one in spite of the fact that in relative terms the number of analysts practicing group psychotherapy has dwindled. Concomitantly, over the past two decades, there has been an explosion in the number of other mental health professionals who swelled the ranks of practicing group therapists. Psychologists, social workers, psychiatric nurses, occupational therapists, counselors, clergymen, and others have moved in to respond to a tremendous need to run groups.

These new professions have brought with them a variety of training and work backgrounds, which lead to such a great diversification of input in terms of ideas and practice that up to date the discipline of group therapy has been unable to integrate it sufficiently. A significant contribution factor leading to this development has been the enormous decentralization of the group psychotherapy scene. This evolution is further attributable to a number of factors: (1) the great variety of theories present, (2) the large geographical distances between centers, (3) the fact that we are not dealing with a quantifiable object, but with a body of knowledge that is also an art, and (4) institutional rivalry.

Sociocultural Factors

Both the theory and the practice of group psychotherapy have been irrevocably influenced by the environment from which it has evolved and in which it has operated. The nonmedical mental health disciplines brought with them broader perspectives beyond the psychoanalytic one. Thus group therapists became increasingly aware of the links between the intrapsychic, the interpersonal and the social functioning of the individual. The interdisciplinary conflicts of earlier times were later replaced by debates focusing on the amount and quality of training that different therapists have acquired. Much of the discomfort had to do with the activities of a variety of self-professed and often minimally trained leaders. That these could establish themselves and often flourish has to do with the disenchantment of a segment of the population with any organized and established treatment modality—or for that matter religion, politics, and moral values in general.

Furthermore, a number of group therapists have promised more than they or anyone else could ever deliver. Group therapy can become a panacea for a troubled society and its members. It is not a substitute for religion, philosophy, and sheer common sense. Group therapy cannot be practiced as a lifestyle. Besides, when political, social, cultural, and moral consensus ceased to exist in our societies, it is unrealistic to expect it to survive intact among group therapists.

An increase in the community's social and psychological awareness and assertiveness has led to a consumer-initiated and consumer-related scrutiny of the whole field of group therapy. With the intention to pacify governments and the public and to avoid recrimination among professionals, peer review committees and continuing educational opportunities have been established. In addition, a definite trend, influenced both by government and society at large, toward standard setting and accreditation in group psychotherapy (as much as in other areas of health care delivery) has gathered momentum.

Personal and Financial Factors

The art component in group psychotherapy has attracted a large number of leaders who have attempted both to rationalize (and at times unwittingly to supplant) their own hypotheses by sheer charisma and personality. The egos of these gurus often transcend regular boundaries and are too inflated to tolerate other theories and approaches. The views of these high priests of group therapy turn into idealogies with which the adherents identify. Orthodoxy and obstinancy in this area can lead to ferociously fought holy wars against the nonbelievers and/or dissidents.

It is worthwhile to remember that not all the acrimony relates to pious matters of postulates and concepts. The group therapy market is lucrative in many places, and intense competition to corner fair parts of it can be one of the tacit motives behind a disagreement on matters of theory.

Orientation

One of the most common and caustic debates in group therapy has been the one between the proponents of two different schools of thought. Others have been generated between the more and the less orthodox adherents of the same theoretical orientation.

At present few claim to represent ideal, comprehensive concepts both for theory and practice. In the age of control groups, duplicability, accountability, efficacy, and cost effectiveness, the focus has shifted to depict one's model as the *least* vulnerable on the above and other criteria. The question now is not whether one has the answer for all patients, but rather how impressive and effective one's representation is in comparison with alternate (and competing) modalities. Increasingly, the ability to offer *specific* treatment methods for clear-cut target problems will become decisive. These definite modalities of intervention become very important at a time when expanding numbers of group therapists and patients realize that there is more than one option from which to choose. Key symptoms are needed to be identified early enough in the evaluation process. Thereafter a referral should be made to the therapist with the most specific approach for the particular problem.

Training

The issue of training is the heraldry of group therapy. One shows one's colors according to the type of training one has received. Trainees are remarkably faithful to their alma mater, and this loyalty explains the intense competition for them. It is therefore of great significance for professional organizations to be able to enforce certain minimal and preferably *uniform standards* of training among their members.

There are many areas of disagreement in regard to what constitutes a well-balanced training program. The major issues involved have been extensively reviewed and discussed in a recent paper by the author (49). Those views will be only summarized here, and some relevant ones critically evaluated.

The eligibility of candidates in terms of their previous professional experience is a thorny subject. While the more traditional training centers require a couple of years of experience in both individual and group psychotherapy, less stringent institutions often accept interest and enthusiasm as adequate prerequisites, without even the need to belong to one of the helping professions. The second group represents a high risk due to a one-sided, narrow theoretical education. In addition, members of this group are more likely to be tempted to make up for their training by charisma alone. Training in such a treatment modality does depend almost exclusively on modeling a particular personality approach that cannot be automatically integrated by every given therapist candidate.

Very few training centers screen a candidate's personality adequately. Yet the character variable is probably the most important factor affecting leadership efficacy in groups (20, 57). This author has advocated for some time that aside from multiple interviews with at least two interviewers present, group therapy candidates should undergo selected projective psychological testing, to exclude those with more severe personality disturbances (49). Each institution could decide where to draw the line in terms of acceptability. This suggestion has generated considerable controversy even among experienced training group therapists. Some have contended that at the beginning all budding therapists exhibit so much psychopathology that hardly any of them would qualify for training. Unfortunately, these teachers postpone decision-making until the candidates are well into their training and at times personal therapy. The responsibility in this respect has to be taken early. An obviously insecure, suspicious, dependent, or hostile/aggressive therapist should not be allowed to proceed in a training program—and *perhaps* be declared incompetent on its completion. It would be unfair to the patients he will have (mis-) treated in the meantime and a disappointment to himself. Furthermore such a permissive approach tends to tarnish the reputation of group therapy as an effective and humane treatment modality.

Much controversy has focused on the advantages of the comprehensively eclectic versus the narrower, more specialized approach in training programs. In the author's opinion, the dilemma is not an either/or issue but rather is to ascertain in what sequence the learning is to be carried out. Beginning therapists should have an exposure to the major schools of thought in group psychotherapy. As they become more experienced they can choose the method most agreeable to them. From that point on the therapist can acquire a special expertise with that technique.

Most training institutes tend to agree in principle as to the desirable components of the program. These usually include lectures, seminars, and reading lists on theory and practice. Another segment comprises individual and/or other supervision, peer group learning, observation of a group run by an experienced leader, and being a therapist in a group. Certainly one is expected to participate as a member of a training or therapy group.

The disputes of this area center primarily on three issues: (1) How large should the experiential portion be in relationship to the cognitive aspects of training? There is no set rule on this subject. However, it is very important to point out that any imbalance of these ingredients is likely to produce therapists with serious deficits either in their theoretical comprehension or in their ability to empathize with individuals in the group and understanding the impact of group dynamics. (2)

Should the candidate undergo personal group psychotherapy in a group with his peers (other trainees) or with bona fide patients? Despite more protective views in some centers, studies by Alnoes and Sigrell, Berger, Mullan and Rosenbaum, Pines, and others lend support to the author's impression that groups composed solely of mental health professionals tend to be overly defensive and intellectualizing (3, 9, 10, 22, 38, 42, 49, 60). (3) Whether didactic or experiential learning should take precedent has not yet been unequivocally decided. There are pros and cons for each, but in practice reality considerations dictate the sequence. Experience of the author with the Ontario Group Psychotherapy Association seems to indicate, though, that trainees might benefit more from the theoretical program after participation in a therapy group.

Training (T-) or study groups have generated a number of provocative thoughts. Are they a personal learning experience or therapy? At times it might be difficult to draw the line and the temptation to slip into therapy is great (49). Nevertheless, there is sufficient evidence (18, 28, 55) to suggest that T-groups are more useful as a vehicle for teaching the importance of group dynamics and interpersonal relations through personal experience in a group.

Furthermore, can T-groups be useful to professionals working at the same place? While it has been maintained by some that it does not matter or that it works as long as the group leader is from an outside institution, too many indicators point to the contrary. One cannot disregard the reality that this group must continue to work together after the T-group experience is over. Yet, if too many negative feelings have been generated, the results can be deleterious, and future cooperation among the team members could be in danger (18).

The use of videotapes in training and therapy has been hailed as a major step for over a decade (1, 2, 9, 54). It can provide an additional source of objective data, by capturing and providing clarification on group dynamics and interpersonal phenomena. In therapy this material can be discussed with resistant patients. In training it provides useful glimpses into the techniques of experienced therapists.

The trouble in practice with this method is that good video sections need considerable editing and extra time for reply and discussion. Thus few patients, therapists, and trainees have the time and resources to use this interesting modality more than sporadically.

Group Size

The number of patients in a given group has been a neglected issue that has contributed its share to the criticism regarding the efficacy of group psychotherapy. Theories in group psychotherapy have derived primarily from observation of individual psychotherapy and small group dynamics, related essentially to functioning neurotic patients. However, group therapy practice has included numerous large ward and milieu groups, composed of much more severely debilitated patients. Thus considerable knowledge has been extrapolated from stable, long-term, cohesive outpatient groups, consisting of six to nine members and a regular therapist (or cotherapist) to institutional groups made up of twenty to thirty patients, with shorter periods of stay and frequent turnovers in members and often in therapists as well. Besides the latter frequently tend to be minimally trained in group psychotherapy. In spite of these basic differences the techniques employed have not been sufficiently adapted and the expectations related to outcome not adjusted accordingly. These gatherings seldom evolve over the early stages of group development and are unable to accomplish the kind of work that accompanies intimacy and individuation. Nevertheless, many professionals have been "turned off" groups by participating in these ill-conceived, floundering, lip-service sessions.

Leaderless Groups

A topic which has vexed a number of innovators has been that of viability of leaderless groups. These are to be differentiated from the alternate meetings, as described by Kadis and Wolf (28, 29), and the occasional sessions in the absence of the therapist, both of which have proved to be quite helpful and therapeutic.

Alternate occasional sessions for patients, either planned on a regular basis or held during the therapist's absence, seem to increase cohesiveness, encourage independence and help giving, stimulate transference, loosen inhibitions, encourage passive patients to become more active, and promote receptivity to peer feedback (5, 26, 52).

The proponents of the regularly leaderless group maintain that they are therapeutic to the patients and useful for group therapists who study process phenomena. Evidence supporting the beneficial effects of these leaderless patient groups is anecdotal (16, 17, 41) and has been viewed by most as unproductive (52). Self-help groups such as Alcoholics Anonymous, Schizophrenics and Neurotics Anonymous, and Recovery Incorporated seem to represent partial exceptions for selected patients.

The evaluation of leaderless groups for experienced therapists is somewhat more positive but equally lacks methodology (23, 24, 30, 31, 39). Furthermore, gains in terms of increase in self-esteem, letting down of defensive barriers, and better understanding of group dynamics occurred only in highly motivated, satisfied, and well-intentioned therapists with low expectations (30, 39). The risks and potential for failure have been manifold. The author's experience with such groups has been reflected in a number of studies. The participants in them tend to be highly resistant, playing the therapist (19, 37), attacking persons not present, projecting negative traits on others, and denying emotional needs (31). As Woods pointed out, there is a strong "narcissistic anxiety inherent in discussing one's clinical work with peers" (61). Open competition with mutual denigration and distrust abound, along with games of "who can interpret best." Many leaderless professional groups have disintegrated over the issue of leadership (25). One gets the impression that while such a peer group can work best with members who are unfamiliar with each other and do not work together, it is a highly overrated modality as a long-term procedure. To quote Borriello "there is no such thing as a leaderless group" (13). The risks and drawbacks in this method of the leaderless group outweigh by far the potential advantages. There is overwhelming evidence in the literature showing that the benefits do not measure up to that of a properly led therapeutic or study group (13, 48, 49, 55, 57, 60).

Composition of Groups

A strong dissonance regarding the optimal composition of therapeutic groups has plagued therapists from the early stages. The argument focuses on the preference of homogeneity versus heterogeneity in the group. The criteria most often mentioned are those of diagnosis, psychodynamics, racial or ethnic origin, social class, sex, sexual orientation, and age. The rationale in decision-making is influenced by sociopolitical, geographical, temporal, personal, and demand-and-supply factors and by purely clinical considerations. A number of authors have suggested that group leaders should strive for maximum heterogeneity in the patients' problem areas and patterns of coping and for homogeneity in the patients' degree of vulnerability and capacity to tolerate anxiety (6, 34, 38, 43, 60). Nevertheless, because of the above factors these recommendations often have not been carried out.

To achieve a group that is relatively conflict free has been the reason for including patients with similar diagnostic entities, for example, neuroses and mild-to-moderate personality disorders. However, in such a group this author often has included one borderline person who would do reasonably well.

On the other hand, the issues of ethnic or racial origin and social class—and the two often overlap—have been a powder keg for the past twenty years. In many regions, therapists would not consider anything but a homogeneous group along the above lines. In fact, often the efficacy of a white, middle-class therapist has been questioned when the group members have dissimilar backgrounds (14, 15). The literature on this topic is difficult to evaluate because much of it is anecdotal or tendentious, and wishful thinking or overcompensated guilt is often substituted for methodical research (14, 15). What seems to be clear is that race, ethnic origin, or social class of both the patients and the therapist *does* affect the outcome of therapy (15). The larger the degree of social and racial polarization in a particular community the more difficult it becomes to work with "mixed" groups. The experience of the author and others in working with groups containing minority members indicates that dealing with the issues of one's sociocultural background *early* in therapy is a prerequisite to the successful functioning of that particular group (14).

A similar approach pertains to homosexual or lesbian group members. Contrary to some other reports, this author found it useful to treat a single representative of an ethnic or sexual preference minority in a "regular" group—taking into account the earlier mentioned precondition.

The exact ratio of men to women is not of great therapeutic

significance. All groups composed solely of men or women, however, are likely to be constricted at the level of interaction and will have an inclination to deal with sexual issues superficially. Furthermore, an important reality aspect of learning how to communicate and behave in a heterosexual society is not given in such a one-sex group (48).

The age limits in an adult group need not be taken too rigidly. As long as one excludes the two extremes, adolescent types of problems or issues of the elderly, the various age groups tend to mix well and foster a gamut of parent-child transferences.

Whether a patient can and should be simultaneously in group and individual therapy—in an ongoing way or when in crisis—depends primarily on the following factors: (1) Is there a real indication for a double-barreled approach? (41, 7, 11, 21, 47, 50, 61). (2) If individual therapy is to be done by someone other than the group therapist, how good is communication likely to be between the two to avoid overlap and acting out? (40). (3) The nature of the individual therapy: it should not run contrary to the group goals and should not confuse the patient with conflicting techniques. Thus pharmacotherapy (32) or behavioral modification is less likely to create difficulties with a patient being in a psychoanalytically oriented group than Gestalt therapy or transactional analysis.

Co-Therapy

Co-therapy has taken the field of group therapy by storm over the past decade. There is considerable literature available (8, 46, 56) to point out the advantages of this set-up to patients and therapists (or trainees). The benefits quoted include an enhancement of the group process, an increase in the level of interaction, a broader screen for a more accelerated transference, a great ability to confront patient resistance, an amplification in the validity and intensity of the interpretations, and a great sensitivity to a wider range of psychological issues. However, while this method has gained wide acceptance and praise for treatment and training purposes, many of the warnings and preconditions required for its successful practice have been largely overlooked. Even the most ardent proponents point out that co-therapy is best employed with special patient populations, such as the distrustful, the patient with the identity problem, the deprived patient, the emotionally labile (56), the homosexual (12, 53), the exhibitionist (36), the psychopath (27), and the obsessive individual (33).

Co-therapy should not be seen as the answer to all patients in group psychotherapy. Certainly its present application and evaluation is too nebulous to stand up to a more thorough investigation. Rosenbaum states that "contrary to popular assumption co-therapy is not an easy technique. It requires considerable maturity on the part of both leaders, and it should be used cautiously with experienced therapists" (46). Furthermore, two therapists do not necessarily provide better treatment than one does. A consensus exists that the nature of the relationship between the co-therapists is *the* vital factor in making such an endeavor work (8, 35, 44, 46, 49, 58). Thus a whole paper by Williams (59) dealt with the contract that co-therapists should work through before starting their group. Sibling rivalry, the potential for "splitting" in the Kleinian sense (51), and status needs have been identified as the biggest risks from the therapist's point of view.

To the above we have to add a special concern regarding the training potential of this modality. The roles of each of the co-therapists have to be defined carefully, and one should not forget that training in co-therapy does not necessarily qualify one to lead a group alone.

Owing to the above insights, a vast literature scrutinizing the pitfalls of co-therapy in group psychotherapy has been collated over the years (35, 45, 46, 49, 58). The greatest risk yet to be dealt with has been elucidated in an excellent review article by Roman and Meltzer (45). These authors have evaluated critically the co-therapy literature—*with specific relevance to treatment results*. Their study points out that most of the reports are of anecdotal nature, addressing themselves primarily to the effect of co-therapy on the group process rather than to therapeutic outcome. Roman and Meltzer stress that nowhere has the specific source of the co-therapists' power or the particular nature of its effects been systematically explored (45). Rosenbaum has been most aware of this preoccupation of "what is in there for the therapist?" by stating that "therapists are not there to treat one another." He goes on to warn that co-therapy techniques may have become more meaningful to therapists than to the patient (46).

Present indications from practice and theory point out that the best constellation in co-therapy is given when the co-leaders are of opposite sex, of different professional disciplines, and of equal status. Future studies are needed to demonstrate to the many patients involved in co-therapy that they are reaping real and not imagined benefits.

Discussion

The purpose of presenting some of these controversies in the field of group psychotherapy has to do with the need to make therapists aware of the pitfalls involved in oversimplifications, generalization, and jumping on a rolling bandwagon, without knowing where it comes from and in which direction it is heading. Group therapy has not benefited from a chaotic free-for-all as far as its professional reputation has been concerned.

This author does not presume to be able to implement changes long overdue. However, he proposes a number of suggestions for consideration: (1) The rules for training in group psychotherapy should be firmed up, and as much as feasible, made uniform in the various centers. The medical model, while under considerable attack for other reasons, can serve to demonstrate how insistence on certain standards allows for cross-regional and cross-country comparison and evaluation of the level of expertise attained. (2) In areas of dispute among group therapists where boundaries between "right" and "wrong" get blurred or are based more on personal factors, compromises that favor primarily the patient's prognosis are indicated. (3) Teachers and supervisors do have a responsibility vis-à-vis their trainees to take informed and judicious stands on dissenting issues. This action would help to reduce confrontations and to promote an understanding of the specificality of various group therapeutic treatment modalities.

References

1. Alger, I., & Hogan, P. The impact of videotape recording on involvement in group therapy. *J. Psychoanal. Groups* 2: 50–56, 1967.

2. Alger, I. Television image confrontation in group therapy. In C. J. Sager & H. Singer Kaplan (eds.), *Progress in Group and Family Therapy*, pp. 135–150. New York: Brunner/Mazel, 1972.

3. Alnoes, R., & Sigrell, B. Evaluation of the outcome of training groups using an analytic group psychotherapy technique. *Psychother. Psychosom.* 25: 168–175, 1975.

4. Argelander, H. Individual psychotherapy and group psychotherapy in combination. *Gruppenpsychother. Gruppendyn.* 8: 141–151, 1974.

5. Astrachan, B. A., Harrow, M., Becker, R. E., Schwartz, A. H., & Miller, J. C. The unled patient group as a therapeutic tool. *Internat. J. Group Psychother.* 17: 178–191, 1967.

6. Bach, G. *Intensive Group Therapy*, New York: Ronald Press, 1954.

7. Battegay, R. Individual psychotherapy and group psychotherapy as single treatment methods and in combination. *Acta Psychiat. Scand.* 48: 43–48, 1972.

8. Benjamin, S., Jr. Cotherapy: A growth experience for therapists. *Int. J. Group Psychother.* 22: (2), 199–209, 1972.

9. Berger, M. M. Experiential and didactic aspects of training in therapeutic group approaches. *Amer. J. Psychiat.* 126: (6), 845–850, 1969.

10. Berman, A. L. Group psychotherapy training: Issues and models. *Small Group Behaviour* 6: (3), 325–344, 1975.

11. Bieber, T. Combined individual and group psychotherapy. In H. Kaplan & B. Sadock (eds.), *Comprehensive Group Psychotherapy*, 153–169. Baltimore: Williams & Wilkins, 1971.

12. Birk, L., Miller, E., & Cohler, B. Group psychotherapy for homosexual men by male-female cotherapists. *Acta Psychiat. Scand. (Suppl.)* 218: 1–36, 1970.

13. Boriello, J. B. Leadership in the therapist centered group-as-a-whole psychotherapy approach. *Internat. J. Group Psychother.* 26: 149–162, 1976.

14. Calnek, M. Racial factors in the counter-transference: The black therapist and the black client. *Amer. J. Orthopsychiat.* 40: 39–46, 1970.

15. Carkhuff, R. R., & Pierce, R. Differential effects of therapist race and social class upon patient depth of self exploration in the initial clinical interview. *J. Couns. Psychol.* 31: (6), 632–634, 1967.

16. Fairweather, G. W. *Social Psychology in Treating Mental Illness: An Experimental Approach*. New York: Wiley, 1964.

17. Freund, R. B. A patients' autonomous society as a method of group psychotherapy. *Psychiat. Quarterly. Suppl.* 33: 317–332, 1959.

18. Gottschalk, L. A., & Pattison, E. M. Psychiatric perspectives on T-groups and the laboratory movement: An overview. *Amer. J. Psychiat.* 126: (6), 823–839, 1969.

19. Grotjahn, M. The qualities of the group therapist. In H. Kaplan & B. Sadock (eds.), *Comprehensive Group Psychotherapy*, pp. 757–773. Baltimore: Williams & Wilkins, 1971.

20. Hartley, D., Roback, H. B., & Abramovitz, S. I. Deterioration effects in encounter groups. In H. B. Roback, S. I. Abramovitz, & D. S. Stransberg (eds.), *Group Psychotherapy Research*, pp. 214–221. Huntington, N.Y.: R. E. Krieger Publishing Co., 1979.

21. Heigl-Evans, A., & Heigl, F. On the combination of psychoanalytic individual and group therapy. *Gruppenpsychother. Gruppendyn.* 8: 97–121, 1974.

22. Hidas, G., & Buda, B. Dynamisches Modell des Wilderstandes in der Ausbildungsgruppe. Ref. III, Internat. Congress. Gruppentherapie, Vienna, Med. Akademie, 1968.

23. Hunt, W., & Issacharoff, A. History and analysis of a leaderless group of professional therapists. *Amer. J. Psychiat.* 132: 1164–1167, 1975.

24. Imber, S., et al. Suggestibility, social class and the acceptance of psychotherapy. *J. Clin. Psychol.* 12: 341–344, 1956.

25. Issacharoff, A., & Hunt, W. Observation on group process in a leaderless group of professional therapists. *Group* 1: 162–171, 1977.

26. Kadis, A. L. The alternate meeting in group psychotherapy. *Amer. J. Psychother.* 10: 275–291, 1956.

27. Kagan, H., & Zucker, A. Treatment of a "corrupted" family by rabbi and psychiatrist. *J. Rel. Health* 9: 22–34, 1970.

28. Kaplan, S. R. Therapy groups and training groups: Similarities and differences. *Int. J. Group Psychother.* 17: 473–504, 1967.

29. Kellerman, H. *Group Psychotherapy and Personality: Intersecting Structures,* pp. 268–297. New York: Grune & Stratton, 1979.

30. Kline, R. M. Dynamics of a leaderless group. *Internat. J. Group Psychother.* 22: 234–242, 1972.

31. Kline, F. M. Terminating a leaderless group. *Internat. J. Group Psychother.* 24: 452–459, 1974.

32. Kymissis, P. Pharmacotherapy combined with analytically oriented group therapy. In L. R. Wolberg, M. L. Aronson, & A. R. Wolberg (eds.), *Group Therapy in 1978*, pp. 131–139. New York: Stratton Intercontinental Medical Book Corp., 1978.

33. Lassiter, R., & Willett, A. B. Interaction of group cotherapists in the multidisciplinary team treatment of obesity. *Int. J. Group Psychother.* 23: 82–92, 1973.

34. Locke, N. *Group Psychoanalysis.* New York: New York University Press, 1961.

35. Maclennan, B. W. Co-therapy. *Int. J. Group Psychother.* 15: 154–166, 1965.

36. Mathis, J., & Collins, M. Mandatory group therapy for exhibitionists. *Amer. J. Psychiat.* 126: 1162–1167, 1970.

37. Morgan, D. W. A note on analytic group psychotherapy for therapists and their wives. *Int. J. Group Psychother.* 21: 244–247, 1971.

38. Mullan, H., & Rosenbaum, M. *Group Psychotherapy: Theory and Practice,* pp. 115–173. New York: The Free Press, 1978.

39. Nobler, H. A peer group for therapists: Successful experience in sharing. *Int. J. Group Psychother.* 30: 51–60, 1980.

40. Ormont, L. R., & Strean, H. S. *The Practice of Conjoint Therapy,* pp. 30–85. New York: Human Sciences Press, 1978.

41. Pettit, W. W. What is an autonomous group? *Autonomous Groups Bulletin* 10: 2–5, 1955.

42. Pines, M. Group Psychotherapy: Frame of reference for training. In W. De Moor & H. R. Wyngaarden (eds.), *Psychotherapy and Training.* Elsevier/North-Holland Biomedical Press, 1980.

43. Powdermaker, F., & Frank, J. *Group Psychotherapy,* pp. 66–112. Cambridge, Mass.: Harvard University Press, 1953.

44. Rabin, H. M. How does co-therapy compare to regular group therapy? *Amer. J. Psycother.* 21: 244–255, 1967.

45. Roman, M., & Meltzer, B. Cotherapy—A review of current literature (with special reference to therapeutic outcome). *J. Sex & Marital Ther.* 3: (1), 63–77, 1977.

46. Rosenbaum, M. Co-therapy. *Comprehensive Group Psychotherapy,* 501–517. Baltimore: Williams & Wilkins, 1971.

47. Sadock, B. Combined individual and group psychotherapy. In A. M. Freedman & A. J. Kaplan (eds.), *Comprehensive Textbook of Psychiatry* (vol. 1, second edition), pp. 1877–1891. Baltimore: Williams & Wilkins, 1975.

48. Salvendy, J. T., & Gruenberger, J. Psychotherapeutische und leistungspsychologische Testerfahrungen in einer Schizophrenengruppe. *Ztshrft, f. Psychotherapie, u. med. Psychologie* 18: (2), 58–66, 1968.

49. Salvendy, J. T. Group psychotherapy training: A quest for standards. *Can. J. Psychiatry* 25: 394–402, 1980.

50. Scheindler, S. & Porter, K. Group Psychotherapy combined with individual psychotherapy. In L. Bellak & B. Karasu (eds.), *Special Techniques in Individual Psychotherapy.* 1980.

51. Segal, H. *Introduction to the Work of Melanie Klein,* New York: Basic Books, 1964.

52. Seligman, M., & Desmond, R. The leaderless group phenomenon: A historical perspective. *Internat. J. Group Psychother.* 25: (3), 277–290, 1975.

53. Singer, M., & Fischer, R. Group psychotherapy for male homosexuals by a male and female cotherapy team. *Int. J. Group Psychother.* 17: 44–52, 1967.

54. Stoller, F. H. Videotape feedback in the group setting. *J. New Ment. Dis.* 148: 457–466, 1969.

55. Taintor, Z. Group sensitivity training for psychiatric residents. *J. Psychiatr. Educ.* 1: 93–99, 1977.

56. Treppa, J., & Nunnelly, K. Interpersonal dynamics related to the utilization of multiple therapy. *Amer. J. Psychother.* 28: (1), 71–83, 1974.

57. Truax, C. B., Carkhuff, R. R., & Kodman, F. Relationships between therapist offered conditions and patient change in group psychotherapy. *J. Clin. Psychol.* 21: 327–329, 1965.

58. Williams, R. A. A contract for co-therapists in group psychotherapy. *J. Psychiat. Nurs. & Ment. Health Services,* 11–14, June 1976.

59. Wolf, A. The psychoanalysis of groups. *Amer. J. Psychother.* 4: 16–50, 1950.

60. Yalom, I. D. *The Theory and Practice of Group Psychotherapy.* New York: Basic Books, 1975.

61. Zander, W. Special conclusion concerning conjoint therapy based on experience with a demonstration group. *Gruppenpsychother. Gruppendyn.* 8: 122–130, 1974.

Is the Law Interfering
with Treatment?

Barry B. Swadron, Q.C., LL.B., LL.M.
Susan G. Himel, LL.B.

Psychiatrists and other treatment personnel have not always been enamoured with the law. Many feel that they should be given *carte blanche* more or less to go about their business as they see it should be done. Some treatment professionals, on the other hand, have bemoaned what they see as a lack of direction or precision in the law. The debate will always flourish. The pendulum swings back and forth, and the law in every given jurisdiction reflects or is about to catch up with the thinking of the times.

There is a growing concern that something has gone wrong in mental health programming in the last decade or so. A number of forces, all with some validity (at least on the surface), have combined to go a long way toward emptying the large, burgeoning mental hospitals as we once knew them. What are these forces? They are the concept of normalization (wanting the disabled to live as others do), the dictation of economic reality (which requires conservation of public funds in times of skyrocketing institutional costs), and the movement toward the recognition of greater civil liberties.

The increasing acceptance of the principles of normalization and deinstitutionalization of the mentally disabled has resulted in the concept of outpatient care assuming a greater role. The trend to outpatient care can be justified only if the community can provide adequate support through services that enable those with disabilities to survive and function. The availability of and ease of admission to institutional care will influence the population that should be served by outpatient programs.

There have been both therapeutic and legal justifications given for the de-institutionalization movement. It has been argued that a patient will benefit from treatment that minimizes his or her removal from the community. The legal arguments focus on the liberty interests of the individual. This paper addresses the question of whether the law, in the context of current mental health programs, is assisting or interfering with the treatment of the mentally handicapped.

Since the 1950s, involuntary civil commitment laws have been the subject of much debate. It has been stated many times that the detention of an individual who has not been convicted of a crime represents the most serious deprivation of liberty in our democratic culture. Some critics, such as Thomas Szasz, have used this argument even to advocate the abolition of involuntary commitment.

In some jurisdictions in Canada and to a greater degree in the United States, the legislative response has been to clarify and restrict the criteria for admission to psychiatric institutions and to increase the procedural protections involved in the commitment process. The tightening of commitment laws has had a direct impact on treatment: where and how it is administered, who receives it and, indeed, whether it is received at all.

Commitment Criteria

Until recently, for example, Ontario legislation authorized the involuntary hospitalization of any person who "suffers from a mental disorder of a nature or degree so as to require hospitalization in the interests of his own safety or the safety of others" and "is not suitable for admission as an informal patient." This test allowed a degree of flexibility and discretion.

Pressure for restriction of the criteria came mainly from the Canadian Civil Liberties Association, which advocated limited discretion of physicians in order to protect the rights of would-be patients. The response of the Ontario legislature was to adopt "serious bodily harm" as the operative criterion for involuntary commitment. *The Mental Health Act* now provides:

8.—(1) Where a physician examines a person and has reasonable cause to believe that the person

(a) has threatened or attempted or is threatening or attempting to cause bodily harm to himself;

(b) has behaved or is behaving violently towards another person or has caused or is causing another person to fear bodily harm from him; or

(c) has shown or is showing a lack of competence to care for himself,

and if in addition the physician is of the opinion that the person is apparently suffering from mental disorder of a nature or quality that likely will result in

(d) serious bodily harm to the person;

(e) serious bodily harm to another person; or

(f) imminent and serious physical impairment of the person,

the physician may make application in the prescribed form for a psychiatric assessment of the person.

The practical effect of this amendment is to make commitment criteria more stringent.

Other Canadian jurisdictions have generally retained less precise standards for commitment, such as "for his own protection or welfare or for the protection of others," a "danger to his own safety or safety of others," and "in the interests of his own safety or the safety of others."

Commitment Procedures

Commitment procedures more clearly differ between Canadian and American jurisdictions. The United States' commitment model generally requires a form of judicial approval of any continued detention, following a brief period of initial confinement. No Canadian jurisdiction currently requires court involvement in the commitment process. Most Canadian jurisdictions proceed with commitment based on the certificate of one or two physicians and require periodic renewals of those certificates. Rights of periodic review by quasi-judicial boards are available by statute.

Special Factors Reducing Institutional Care

In the United States, certain factors stand out in explaining the reduced inpatient populations resulting in greater numbers requiring management on an outpatient basis. There is a development of the concept of the right to be treated in the least restrictive setting, which flows from the judicial recognition of the premise that confinement can only be sustained if accompanied by adequate treatment. There has also been the judicial creation of standards for the quality of care and development of environments with superior treatment programs resulting in higher health costs. For example, following the leading decision of *Wyatt v. Stickney*, which set out a detailed list of standards for Alabama mental institutions, the population in those institutions was drastically reduced although the costs of institutional care increased. Additionally, the constitutional right to adequate treatment in a humane environment has resulted in the necessary investigation of noninstitutional settings as alternatives.

For better or for worse, Canada has not been confronted with these "special factors"—at least, not yet. There have been two major criticisms directed at the restricted use of mental institutions. One is that de-institutionalization is really a pragmatic method of reducing expenditures. The second is that the focus on individual liberty interests has taken attention away from the real problem, which is shortage of treatment. It is important to protect the person from unnecessary coercive treatment, but the rhetoric in this area allows the real problem of the insufficiency of available treatment to be masked. Could it be that the civil libertarian perspective is not disliked by governments because it allows for reduced expenditures?

Consequences of De-Institutionalization

The trend to de-institutionalization has occurred rapidly, with a sharp decline in patients resident in mental hospitals. However, the difficult process of building adequate community services has occurred slowly and there is evidence it is sadly lacking. In the words of Mechanic (1976):

Even a cursory examination of the present state of affairs shows an enormous gap between the ideology and realities of community care. While it has been relatively simple to alter administrative policies to avoid hospitalization and to release hospitalized patients as quickly as possible, the development of an adequate framework of community services to assist the mentally ill or their families has been very slow. As economic pressures have mounted for federal and state governments, as well as for localities, there has been less willingness to invest the resources to meet, even minimally, the needs of patients in the community, and the new neighborhood health centers have frequently avoided the most impaired patients. Disturbed and disabled patients are kept in the community under the banner of community care only to suffer community "institutionalism." Various agencies, each attempting to protect its budget, shift the responsibilities to others, leaving many patients greatly in need, unattended and living under appalling conditions.

Facilities that are found for de-institutionalized people are located typically in high population density and low income neighborhoods where community residences are created inexpensively in older, larger homes. Ex-patients find themselves without financial and social resources and without proper supervision and treatment in many cases. There are growing numbers of mentally ill persons functioning at low levels in the community and suffering from personal and social problems. With the cutbacks and limited budgets of community and welfare agencies, the quality of care of those requiring treatment is diminished.

While the conditions that existed in large institutions were less than exemplary, the trend to community care and away from civil commitment should not be an excuse for abdicating responsibility for ensuring that adequate services are available.

Schull (1977) describes the situation as follows:

Excluded from the more desirable neighbourhoods by zoning practices and organized community opposition, the decarcerated deviants are in any case impelled by economics—the need for cheap housing and to be close to a welfare office—to cluster in the ghettos and the decaying core of the inner city. As for the criminal, he is also attracted by the tokenism of police operations in these areas and by the willingness of the wider society to leave ghetto residents to fend for themselves. Decarceration thus forms yet one more burden heaped on the backs of those who are most obviously the victims of our society's inequities. And it places the deviant in those communities least able to care for or cope with him.

The trend to de-institutionalization and reintegration in the community has received much publicity of late as patients discharged with prescriptions of drugs have formed their own "psychiatric ghettoes" in low-cost boarding houses, supported by welfare assistance.

Zoning Restrictions and the Right to Live in the Community

The nineteenth century saw the creation of large, remote, secure institutions for the mentally disabled. Twentieth-century zoning laws fostered the notion of creating pleasant places for "normal" people to live and had the effect of excluding threatening, dissimilar people from such neighborhoods. The preservation of the character of districts as "better residential areas" was considered a legitimate purpose.

Although the idea of community care may be based historically, its widespread support has essentially been taking effect only since the 1950s. With the rationale that "normalization," that is, the availability of patterns and conditions of life as close as possible to norms of mainstream society, the right of the mentally disabled to reside in the community is an issue now at the forefront. The further factors of use of drug therapy resulting in reduced average length of stay of hospital confinement, the research tending to show the destructive effect of institutionalization, and the fiscal advantages to reducing institution populations have contributed to the need for acceptance of the mentally ill in the community. Some legal frameworks have also encouraged community living through recognition of the principle of right to treatment in the least restrictive setting; high standards for institutional care have resulted in the necessity of seeking alternative residential settings.

Although community treatment is desirable, few jurisdictions have developed adequate procedures for monitoring de-institutionalization policies and implementing them. A major obstacle that has interfered with the establishment of community residential facilities is zoning laws. Zoning is the systematic regulation and control of the use and development of real property by, most often, municipal governments. Land use control is done through the division of municipalities into districts. Typically, zoning bylaws prohibit any use except "permitted" uses that generally include classifications such as residential, commercial, and industrial zones. Further subclassifications of residential zones into single-family housing, duplexes, multiple-family dwellings, apartments, boarding homes, and nursing homes are common.

Zoning laws are aimed at separating incompatible uses of adjoining lands to ensure general welfare through restrictions on the full exploitation of an individual owner's property. In consequence, certain groups are excluded from particular residential areas.

The often mentioned concerns of those who seek to exclude community residences for the disabled are: fear of exposure to crime and social deviancy, disturbance of neighborhoods by transients, inadequate supervision of the disabled, and the resulting reduction of property values. The other side of the coin is, of course, the rehabilitative effect of creating homelike, family atmospheres for persons who are in need.

The Definition of "Family" in Zoning Bylaws

Typical restrictive bylaws broadly define "family" as a single housekeeping unit, related by bonds of blood, marriage, and consanguinity. Certain jurisdictions define "family" to include unrelated persons maintaining a single, housekeeping unit. Where single-family dwellings are the only permissible uses in residential areas, community-type residences are accordingly excluded.

The broad definition of "family" has not remained unchallenged. In the United States, in the leading case of *Village of Belle Terre* v. *Boraas*, the Supreme Court considered the constitutionality of an ordinance defining "family" to include any number of related persons but only two unrelated persons living and cooking together. This case involved six unrelated college students who leased a house in a Long

Island village zoned exclusively for single-family dwellings. The Court held that the ordinance was a rational means of achieving the legitimate objective of preserving a "quiet place where yards are wide, people few and motor vehicles restricted." The situation is typical of the problems the nontraditional family faces with most zoning bylaws.

However, certain jurisdictions in the United States have held that where community residences are state-run and approved and funded, local boards do not have the authority to construe an ordinance to exclude group homes. Inconsistent approaches have resulted as those closer to the "family" model may succeed, but groups such as drug users or emergency hostel facilities will not. For example, in *City of White Plains* v. *Ferraioli*, the New York Court of Appeals distinguished the *Belle Terre* case where a defendant leased a building in a single-family district and a nonprofit agency was authorized to operate such group homes under state law. Here, a "family" of a couple, their two children, and ten foster children (seven of whom were siblings) was permitted to continue its operation. The court considered the municipality exceeded its jurisdiction by defining family so narrowly as to exclude a stable group home occupied by persons unrelated in a biological sense. The state of the law seems to be that where a housekeeping situation parallels a "family" set-up, a municipal ordinance will not prevent its existence in a particular zone.

In Canada, the Supreme Court has gone even further. In the recent decision of *Bell* v. *The Queen*, the court dealt with a bylaw that sought to prevent unrelated people from living together by defining "family" in terms of bonds of consanguinity, blood, marriage, or legal adoption. Here, three unrelated males were residing in a house zoned as a single-family dwelling. Their arrangement involved a mutual sharing of expenses with no commercial profit or structural changes to the premises. The argument of the municipality was that such bylaws exist to preserve "better residential districts."

It was held by the Supreme Court of Canada that the bylaw was *ultra vires* the municipality as it sought to create "land zoning by people zoning." It was considered an excess of authority to define "family" in the sense of "related persons" and restrict uses to those who fall within its definition. Perhaps the effects of this case are to open the door to community residential facilities in all areas across the land.

Where Do They Go from Here?

Now that we have brought into the community great numbers of the disabled, we are bound to sort out their residential placements. Surely we must have them residentially settled, as a first measure, before we worry about their treatment and other problems. Unfortunately, it seems not an unnatural tendency for property owners and elected local officials who represent them to want to exclude the dissimilar from their neighborhoods. The not unpredictable allegation of local officials is to blame provincial or state authorities for "dumping" the disabled on them with little warning and the offer of limited resources. Friction is created among municipalities when each blames the other for their "closed door policies." It is becoming more and more evident that provincial or state governments are going to have to intervene, if necessary, by legislating to ensure that each municipality and community takes its fair share of the disabled. The ways and means of accomplishing this end should, to the degree possible, be such that they endeavor to accommodate all interests. Some interests will necessarily be sacrificed or concessions made. There is no other way!

Some specific solutions include qualifying group homes or community residences as a "family use"; deeming such facilities as being a permitted use; allowing special exceptions through spot zoning or issuing conditional use permits; or granting of licenses based upon need, standards, programming, and other factors without reference to any zoning restrictions.

Community Living: Legal Impediments to "Normalization"

The development of the law reflects the great difficulty society has in reconciling two concepts. First, there is the notion that the mentally handicapped should, whenever possible, be treated as their "normal" counterparts. Second, there is the effort to ensure that the mentally handicapped can cope and live reasonably in the midst of other members of society, but to do so effectively, they require supervision and protection. While the creation of special status may be desirable at times, the status will set them apart from others.

An examination of certain laws embracing various fields of human endeavor as they are applied to or affect mentally disabled persons living in the community discloses that there are often competing interests. In an effort to protect the disabled, there is a risk of over-protection that will result in not enabling them to do what others can do. On the other hand, to respect totally the "normalization" concept is to be in peril of failing to protect adequately or even at all. The most I can do in this paper is simply to touch on some areas of endeavor.

Exercising the Franchise

Voting is considered a basic right of democracy. While regulation of the right to vote is a matter that is generally the subject of legislation and varies from one jurisdiction to another, there do exist exclusions in respect to the mentally handicapped. Many of these exclusions are geared to hospitalization and, accordingly, the right to vote is not often subtracted in the case of the mentally disabled living in the community. Some election laws do, however, prohibit persons who are declared mentally incompetent from voting without reference to institutionalization. The rationale for any exclusion from voting on the basis of mental disability is a losing exercise in logic.

Making a Will

Making a will is an essential element of planning one's affairs. The law requires that in order to make a valid will one must have testamentary capacity. If capacity is successfully attacked, a will can be set aside. The tests for determining capacity involve: an understanding of the nature of the act, comprehending that the act is a testamentary disposition; memory and comprehension of the nature of the extent of the estate; comprehension and appreciation of the claims of people who normally should be objects of the bounty; and judgment to make dispositions with understanding and reason.

The rationale for protecting the mentally handicapped in making wills is to prevent undue influence or susceptibility to pressure by others so that the free will of the testator is unfettered. One measure that might avoid the successful attacking of a will would be to append to it a psychiatric report relating to capacity of the testator at the time of its execution. With more and more mentally handicapped in the community, there is a chance that more of them will make wills than before and the frequency of attacking their wills may increase.

Capacity to Sue

A further situation restricting the mentally ill involves the right of an individual to be a party to a civil action, that is to apply to the court for relief. The rationale against an unrestricted right to launch actions has been that the mentally handicapped might be unable to assert their rights appropriately and exercise good judgment in the processing of their actions. Accordingly, where a person of "unsound mind" wants to sue, if he/she has been adjudged mentally incompetent by a court of law he/she must sue by a legal representative such as a "committee." If he/she has not been found incompetent by a court of law but is of "unsound mind," he/she must sue by "next friend" who is appointed by the court to look after the interests of the handicapped individual and instruct counsel on his/her behalf. The actual rules governing the situation may differ according to the jurisdiction.

Right to Education and Training

The mentally ill, emotionally disturbed, and mentally retarded have traditionally been treated and "educated" in large residential institutions or at least in segregated classes or workshops. The effect has been for local schools to feel they are no longer responsible for such individuals. The trend to de-institutionalization raises the important question of who is responsible for training or educating this group to bring them more toward independent living.

The rights of "handicapped" to attend appropriate programs in their public school has been recognized in the United States under the *Education for All Handicapped Children Act* (1975), which was fully implemented in 1978. Canada has not yet reached that stage. It must be remembered, however, that without adequate facilities, staff, and financial resources, mandatory legislation has but a hollow meaning.

Employability and Employment

Legislative provisions creating programs for assistance in training the disabled are fundamental to the goal of successful outpatient therapy. Vocational rehabilitation programs exist in Canada to provide restoration, training, and employment placement for "disabled persons" who because of physical or mental impairment are incapable of pursuing regularly any substantially gainful occupation. While the law is designed to achieve "normalization," the interpretation of the law is strict in that often some are excluded on the basis that their capacity is too low for them to take advantage of programs; that the likelihood of achieving specific vocational goals in the imminent future must be made out; that if the disability is psychiatrically based, the prospects of modification of the problem must be such that they are capable of correction within a "reasonable period of time."

The interpretation of the laws is often influenced by tight budgets and financial constraints in such training programs. In terms of eventual employment, many handicapped individuals find themselves in sheltered workshops segregated from the rest of society. In Ontario, the *Human Rights Code* does not deal with discrimination in refusing employment by reason of physical or mental disability. Often, persons suffering from mental illness were practicing or wished to enter certain professions or occupations and were hindered by the law. Statutes governing the practice of professions and trades often provide for cancellation or suspension of privileges in the event of mental disability. While the object may be to protect the public and the individual from liability for actions related to his/her disability, the terms for loss of the right to practice for "improper conduct," "unfitness," or "incapacity" may be vague and unduly broad. Where such laws exist, the right to a hearing to meet the allegations, procedure for reinstatement, and an assurance that the criteria for incapacity are related to the ability to practice are most important.

The Right to Marry

In Canada, there is both federal and provincial jurisdiction dealing with marriage of residents. The provinces under the guise of regulating licensing and solemnization of marriage have enacted legislation that deals with the capacity of persons to marry. License issuers and persons solemnizing marriages are prohibited from doing so in the case of, for example, the "mentally ill" or "mentally defective." The problem with such legislation is who is to determine the competency of the party seeking to be married? Such laws exist in a vacuum that allows for the most liberal or narrow interpretation depending on the discretion of the license issuer or person solemnizing the marriage.

Since capacity to marry involves an ability to understand the significance and nature of the marriage contract and an appreciation of the responsibilities that flow therefrom, if capacity is lacking, a marriage is invalid and will be annulled if there was no real consent to the marriage. A heavy onus of proof is required to establish that a marriage was void *ab initio*.

Operating a Motor Vehicle

Many view driving a car as a vital part of daily living. In some instances, it amounts to the livelihood of an individual. It stands to reason that many psychiatric patients living in the community will want to drive. At the same time, it is essential that the public be protected from those who are not "fit to drive" on psychiatric grounds. Some jurisdictions impose a legislative duty upon physicians to report to the licensing authorities persons whom they believe unfit to drive on medical grounds. While this procedure makes sense, it will be fair only if the authorities make their decisions on appropriate and reasonable bases.

Concern about Abuse of Criminal Law

Often the criminal law is resorted to where help cannot be obtained for individuals through the health field either due to more stringent civil commitment tests, lack of available services, or unwillingness on the part of the mentally disabled to participate voluntarily. Charges such as assault, harassment, intimidation, or threatening have typically been laid as a means to compel treatment of the mentally ill. In fact, the *Criminal Code* of Canada provides that where an accused person, on the basis of a report or evidence of a physician appears to be suffering from mental illness, the court may remand him for observation for a period of up to thirty or sixty days. Upon court order such individuals are placed in psychiatric hospitals involuntarily for observation (not for treatment). Thereafter, they are returned to court with a psychiatric report indicating fitness to stand trial, whether they are certifiable under the mental health laws, whether they are a danger to themselves or others, and if they are good candidates for probation or bail.

Without going into a further discussion of the criminal law, it seems totally unwarranted to use the criminal process to deal with a person who is sick simply because the mental health laws have failed him/her. This point is not to suggest that there should be immunity given to the mentally disordered from criminal prosecution but, rather, that deeper thought be given to those cases where the problem is really medical and not criminal.

Consent

The common law establishes the inviolability of the person by giving individuals the right to accept or reject treatment. The traditional role of consent has been as a defense against allegations of assault and battery. The classic statement of the basic principle involved is that of Judge Cardozo in *Schloendorff* v. *Society of New York Hospitals*; "Every human being of adult years and sound mind has a right to determine what shall be done with his own body; and a surgeon who performs an operation without his patient's consent commits an assault for which he is liable in damages."

The Canadian courts have accepted this principle and adopted the position that a physician cannot overrule the decision of the patient and submit him/her to procedures to which he/she did not give valid consent; if he/she does so, he/she will be liable even if no negligence or want of skill is shown.

The law of consent has been and, for some time to come, will be a gnawing problem to the mental health professional. Institutional practitioners have wrestled with these difficulties and still must do so. Now the same problems are being increasingly confronted in the community by practitioners who are less familiar with whatever guidelines, however chaotic, that are adopted in the institutional setting. My sympathy goes to those who are working in this field with the hope that somehow and sometime the law of consent will become settled and meaningful.

Sterilization

The laws that have developed regarding sterilization have created problems for the physician involved in psychiatric practice. It is often the case that the parents or guardians of an individual who is incompetent to give valid consent believe that sterilization is necessary to keep the individual in the community. The recent Canadian case of *In the Matter of "Eve"* (1979) has raised real doubts about the validity of such a procedure. The Supreme Court (Family Division) of Prince Edward Island held that the consent of the mother on behalf of her incompetent daughter was insufficient to authorize a nontherapeutic sterilization. The implication of this case is that, absent specific statutory authority, incompetent persons simply may not be sterilized for contraceptive purposes. While it is important to ensure that the mentally handicapped are not subjected to sterilization for inappropriate reasons, a complete prohibition may result in the institutionalization of individuals who might otherwise be able to remain in the community.

The Ontario Ministry of Health is in the process of developing legislation that would create a procedure whereby the nontherapeutic sterilization of incompetent persons could be authorized. Their most recent proposal would require the authorization of a multidisciplinary board before a nontherapeutic sterilization could be performed on an incompetent patient. The board would not be authorized to approve the operation unless the criteria set out in the act or regulations were met.

Abortion

Although there has been a great deal of public discussion on the subject of the availability of abortion in Canada, it is clear that nothing in the *Criminal Code* nor in the traditional common law gives a pregnant woman the absolute right to have her pregnancy terminated. If a mentally disabled person is unable to practice any method of contraception, and sterilization is not possible due to consent requirements, an unwanted pregnancy becomes a real possibility. This event raises the possibility of forcing parenthood on an individual who is incapable of assuming the responsibilities involved.

To carry out a legal therapeutic abortion in Canada, a hospital committee must decide whether the particular case falls within the criterion that the continuation of the pregnancy would or would not be likely to endanger the woman's life or health. No guidelines have been established by Parliament as to the meaning of either the word "endanger" or the word "health," but the words have been considered to be strictly medical. "Health" as a medical term is wide enough to include physical health, mental health, and psychological health. An abortion therefore could be authorized when to allow the mentally disabled person to have the child would result in psychiatric or psychological difficulties. The issue of consent, however, may stick out like a sore thumb, and either it will have to be glossed over (as I suspect it is) or Parliament will have to come to the rescue.

Social Benefits

Many people served by psychiatric outpatient programs will be unable to engage in fully remunerative employment. In order to survive in the community, these people will need to receive more than quality treatment: they also will require some type of financial assistance. The difficulty in designing an appropriate social assistance system for the mentally disabled is in ensuring an adequate income for those who need it without creating a disincentive for the individuals to care for themselves.

The function of government in this area is a most delicate one and one that requires constant monitoring to achieve an appropriate balance.

Guardianship

Typically, in many jurisdictions, where someone is admitted to a psychiatric hospital for treatment, a determination is made whether or not he/she is competent to manage his/her property affairs. Often by legislation, a statutory "committee" is appointed to conserve and protect the patient's assets while he/she is in the facility or identified with it; such protection is relatively simple. Competency will be assessed in light of the nature of assets and effect of the mental disability on their management.

The issue of the competency of the mentally disabled resident in the community to manage their financial affairs is becoming more prominent. While there are court proceedings available to provide for the appointment of "committees" through mental incompetency proceedings so that protection of property may be achieved, such proceedings are often expensive, cumbersome, and slow. Furthermore, the thrust of these types of proceedings is mainly directed to incapacity to manage financial affairs as opposed to protection of the person. What about the questions of consent to medical treatment if capacity is lacking, admission to therapy, rehabilitation and training programs, residential placement and transfer, agreements with social agencies for vocational and education services, and litigation matters relating to the person? Surely these are of great importance in terms of ensuring successful treatment of those in community residential settings.

It has been suggested that a concept of guardianship should be statutorily created to facilitate management and treatment of the mentally handicapped in much the same way as children are protected by child welfare laws. The *Dependent Adults Act* in the

Province of Alberta establishes a residual duty in a public guardian (of the person) to exercise powers in the best interests of dependent adults and in such a way as to encourage dependent adults to become capable of caring for themselves. Those interested in the area should read this very progressive piece of legislation. The law as it stands now in many jurisdictions does not assist either the practitioner or the patient with the support measures necessary to achieve successful outpatient treatment.

Need for Action

The law generally lags behind need. This occurrence appears to be the case in respect of the problems created by the sharply escalating numbers of mentally disabled community residents. Their suffering is so obvious that even to the lay person it is clear that resources must be made available to meet their needs. One of their needs is the existence of appropriate laws and fair application of those laws so that the law fosters and does not interfere with treatment.

References

Alberta *Dependent Adults Act*, S.A. 1976, c. 63.

Bell v. The Queen, 98 D.L.R. (3d) 255 (1979).

City of White Plains v. Ferraioli, 34 N.Y. 2d 300, 313 N.E. 2d 756, 357 N.Y. S. 2d 449 (1974).

Criminal Code, R.S.C. 1970, c. C-34, as amended.

Education for All Handicapped Children Act, 1974 (Pub. L.) 94–142.

"Eve", In the Matter Of (1979) P.E.I. S.C. (Fam. Div.) as yet unreported.

Mechanic, D. Judicial Action and Social Change. In S. Golann, & W. J. Fremouw (eds.), *The Right to Treatment for Mental Patients*. New York: John Wiley & Sons, 1976.

Ontario *Human Rights Code*, R.S.O. 1970, c. 318.

Ontario *Mental Health Act*, R.S.O. 1970, c. 269, s. 8(1) as amended by S.O. 1978, c. 50.

Schloendorff v. Society of New York Hospitals, 211 N.Y. 125 at 129 (1914).

Schull, A. *Decarceration*. Englewood Cliffs, N.J.: Prentice-Hall, 1977.

Village of Belle Terre v. Boraas, 416 U.S. 1 (1974).

Vocational Rehabilitation of Disabled Persons Act, R.S.C. 1970, c. V-7, s. 2.

Wyatt v. *Stickney*, 325 F. Supp. 781, (M.D. Ala. 1971) 334 F. Supp. 1341 (M.D. Ala. 1971), 334 F. Supp. 373, 387 (M.D. Ala. 1972), aff'd. in part, remanded in part, rescinded in part, sub. nom. *Wyatt* v. *Aderholt*, 503 F. 2d 1305 (5th Cir. 1974).

The authors gratefully acknowledge the research assistance of David R. Draper, B.A., LL.B.

On Adding Insight to Injury: Dynamics of Aging

Jack Weinberg, M.D.

May I introduce myself to you. I am seventy years of age and thus am a marked man. My face, my hands, and all of my body parts which are significant in social communication have unmistakably become engraved with age. Before I even uttered a word I have already identified myself to you as a person who occupies an extreme position in the life cycle. My very appearance tempts you to place me within a certain type of perspective. Should my words and actions also betray those features that we, both you and I, associate with advanced age, then you are encouraged to mark me down as one who is strikingly different from you.

However, those surface markings do not tell the entire story. They provide only the background and props. Many are the slings and arrows that assail the body and outrageous fortunes that sere the human soul. Deeply imbedded within me are the joys and sorrows of a life lived. Not only the pain sustained but the continued hope for a life meaningfully lived. My chronological age is but a segment devised by human effort, to deny by its brevity the hundreds of years experienced through the process of cognition emotions. Once having perceived the outer trappings and all of the data extracted from my passport, what is it that you really know about me? Not knowing my inner life, my inner legend, what stereotype may you form about me?

That indeed is the vexing issue that faces me and all those who have reached that period in life that the poets call the *threshold of old age*. It is to the viewing of the inner life of the elderly that I would like to address myself—but then I find myself tongue-tied and humble, for others have done it much earlier and undoubtedly more elegantly. For it is not as if the elderly and their lives have suddenly burst on the scene. True, there are more of us, thus quantitatively more of us have

been narcissistically wounded, but one may question whether
qualitatively.

For centuries they have told us who they are, who they were, and
their legends of the past, not in epic terms but in "flakes of colorful
minutiae" and in allegorical allusions. Philosophers, poets, play-
wrights, and novelists have not avoided speculating and writing with
a depth of psychological insights on this poignant and absorbing life
segment. Add to the above biographies, autobiographies, journals,
last wills and testaments, and the literature is immense. We have been
deluged by this literature, but if we have not listened, why is it that we
have not? Could it be that we have not looked upon this vast accumulated knowledge as scientific data assembled in one or two laborato-
ries and compared to a cohort of controls? Is it because these are
discrete and unique experiences that could not be replicated and
therefore scientifically not valid?

Yet therein lies life's preciousness and reality—for *no life is lived
exactly as another.* Nevertheless, this great variance, as varied in
number as there are human beings, has not inhibited the recording
and theorizing observers from ascribing characteristics to hosts of
groups and eventually to all the elderly alive. Listen and you shall
hear:

Aristophanes (445?–?380 B.C.) was the first to point to the regressive aspects of aging in his famous but by now discredited aphorism:
"Old age is but a second childhood." He spoke of the hostility and
fear of the young for the lechery and impotence of the old. He
recognized that younger men were afraid of ending up like the old,
with sexual desires but no power to gratify them. The young,
Aristophanes thought, fear the old as sexual rivals because they have
wealth, status, and therefore power.

The Greek poet Menander (343?–?291 B.C.) had this to say: "A
long life is a painful thing. O burdensome old age! You have nothing
good to offer mortals, but you are lavish with pain and disease. And
yet we all hope to reach you and we do our very best to succeed."
Aristotle (384–322 B.C.) described the aged as mean, paranoid, ill-
natured, fearful, and pessimistic. "They always expect things to turn
out badly because of their experience of life . . . they live more upon
memory than hope."

Plato (427?–347 B.C.) on the other hand regarded age as freeing man from the slavery of his instincts, thus permitting serenity and the study of philosophy. He has Socrates address Cephalus:

"There is nothing I like better, Cephalus, than conversing with aged men; for I regard them as travellers who have gone a journey which I too may have to go, and of whom I ought to inquire whether the way is smooth and easy, or rugged and difficult. And this is a question I should like to ask of you who have arrived at that time which the poets call the 'threshold of old age.' Is life harder towards the end, or what reports do you give of it?"

"I will tell you, Socrates, what my own feeling is. Men of my age flock together, we are birds of a feather, as the old proverb says. At our meetings the tale of my acquaintances commonly is: 'I cannot eat, I cannot drink, the pleasures of youth and love are fled away. There was a good time once, but now it is gone and life no longer is life.' Some complain of slights put upon them by relatives, others tell you sadly of the many evils their old age causes them. But to me, Socrates, these complainers blame that which is not really at fault. For if old age were the cause, I too (being old) and every other old man would have felt as they do. But this is not my experience, nor that of others whom I have known. . . .

"The truth, Socrates, is that these regrets and complaints about relatives are to be attributed to the same cause, which is not old age, but men's characters and tempers. For he who is of a calm and happy nature will hardly feel the pressure of age; but to him who is of the opposite disposition, youth and age are equally burdensome."

Cicero (106–43 B.C.) too came to the defense of old age. A "blessed impotence" preserved old men from the passions and vices, compensated for by the pleasures of the table, conversation, study, literature, and farming. He like Plato saw the faults of old age not as a result of the weight of years but rather as a result of faulty character.

What is fascinating is that Plato and Cicero ascribe the problems attendant to old age as being characterological and of the "nature" of the human being, neither at that point defining "character" or "nature," while to Aristotle the aged "turn out badly because of their experiences of life!"

The early Hebrew literature does not provide us with any psychological insights into the mysteries of old age. It rather asks for honor, compassion, and understanding for all the old. "Cast me not off in time of old age when my strength fails, forsake me not," says the Psalmist, while Ben-Sirah, in the Apocrypha adds a motif of self-interest: "Dishonor not the old; we shall all be numbered amongst them." The Talmud with great delicacy and concern has a code for understanding and working with the psychologically impaired old: "Even the old man who has forgotten his learning must be treated tenderly, for have not the broken tablets been placed in the Ark of the Covenant side by side with the whole ones."

Respect, acceptance, understanding, and love are the age-old admonitions to man in his conduct to the aged. There is little else that modern psychiatry can add to the above prescription. What we can do above all is to provide an understanding, adding insight to injury so as to alleviate suffering. What then are the highways and byways that crowd the tapestry of the inner life of the old? Let me count the ways, for to speak of old age is to tell stories.

Sir Winston Churchill on his seventieth birthday was honored by his peers, so the story goes, at an elaborate banquet held at the storied Westminster Hall. During the ceremony, a toast with his favorite brandy was made by the master of ceremonies, who said, "We all know that next to his cigars Winston loves this brandy most. In fact, if all the brandy that Winston had consumed were to be poured into this hall, it would more than half fill it!" Whereupon Sir Winston looked at the imaginary line drawn by the speaker, lifted his eyes to the lofty rafters and said, "So much to do and so little time in which to do it! However I shall have a go at it!"

Whether true or apocryphal, what shone through this delightful tale was the indomitable spirit of a septuagenarian to whom life, despite age, was a challenge to be lived fully and consistently, and yet he felt ready for adaptive change.

When faced with the issue of being or nonbeing, the dilemma is resolved in becoming in true Hegelian theoretical formulation of the "unity of opposites" so familiar to us in our clinical work. Continued growth, that is the essense of living.

Shortly after his seventieth birthday, E. B. White made the following comment: "I gaze into the faces of our senior citizens in our Southern cities and they wear a sad look that disturbs me. I am sorry for all those who have agreed to grow old. I haven't agreed yet. Old age is a special problem for me because I've never been able to shed the mental image I have of myself—a lad of about 19."

Wilma Donohue at age seventy gave this view of herself: "I have more measure of feeling about aging when I see the people I was young with, at the university, and all of a sudden I see them in the version of old people. I may not have seen them for a long time, and then I see them after they've stepped over the threshold and are now looking old. I have never thought of them as older people and suddenly I see them as old and I gather a sense of their being different, and I have thought about this. To them, just like I am to myself, there is a consistent personality. I don't recognize that I was 20, 30, 40, 50, 60 and so forth. I just seem to be a consistent personality that's lived a whole life. I realize I look the same to them as they look to me. As far as my feeling is concerned, I don't have that sense. I have the same sense of being a whole person with spirit and interests that are consistent with my life."

She showed so little concern with the outer self but an awareness of an "increased interiority" as Neugarten calls it. This interiority wastes very little time of the added free time of later years, to preoccupation with dissatisfactions, which in turn issue out of an incomplete experience of living.

These are but a few of many examples of self-imagery that older persons have about themselves. Such imagery allows them to lead independent lives, for it is lived on a continuum for a certain perceived level that began earlier in their existence.

The development of a self-image is a dual process, dependent as it is on mechanisms deeply ingrained in one's intrapersonal forces, which mold the perception of the self, and on one's circumambience, social, psychological, and cultural, which helps shape, polish, constrain, and modify the percept of the self.

An American begins life with an "all possible" premise. Anyone can attain the presidency of the United States. Dreams of glory are part of the human experience from earliest childhood. These are nurtured by the gradual acquisition of mastery and by the parental ambitions for their progeny and assurance to them that if they so desire, any goal could be attained. The individual, in whom the dreams of the family have been reposited, never quite loses the held-out promise despite his inability to achieve it.

These dreams, then, lead to emerging behavioral patterns that are bound to inner secret legends that each person carries within. As psychiatrists, we are engaged in a type of life review of each of our patients. The life review permits us to perceive the lifestyle, or more often the life-theme, of the individual (as Binswanger calls it). The life-theme of a person, as an example, may be that of emptiness and a constant search for the fulfilling of the self, as one may encounter in an extremely dependent and/or depressed character. What is not so apparent, even to the astute observer, is the personal legend, as I like to call it, which pervades our being and motivates our behavior. It is tempting to use the term "legend," for in most if not all people, the concept of the self as a dynamic force, interacting with the environment, is, more often than not, tinged with wish rather than reality. It is thus distorted and obscured. The legend leads to a romanticizing of the self and a poetic interpretation of reality that arouses skepticism and even hostility toward the holder of the dream. There are, therefore, personal realities that transcend the obvious truth.

The tragedy of late life, then, is that the legend is running out, and the forces marshaled against the maintenance of an assured image are numerous and often compelling.

Human beings are biopsychosocial creatures. As such they have three ultimate needs: individual well-being and longevity; social alliances and hierarchies necessary for group survival; and the need to seek existential significance. Theirs is a system spiraling constantly to levels of more organized complexity, meaning of course, more differentiated emotions, cognitions, and patterns of transaction. It is this differentiation to which they aspire that fashions people into a unique subsystem within a suprasystem. All components of the suprasystem tend to mold the human being into a conformity congruent with its ordained order and to discourage individual uniqueness and thus, more often than not, are injurious to the free human spirit if not the physical self. The injuries that life deals to the individual are practically inevitable and inexplicable to him/her. His/her interpretation of events may or may not be faulty; his/her need for understanding and insights into behavior and meaning of existence is compelling. To suffer injury in a state of innocence is doubly difficult and unnerving.

Again, my theme is that there are realities that transcend the truth.

Paradoxical though this may seem, it is not so to anyone who has heard the words of the emotionally ill . . . the poetry of the anguished mentality that becomes its credo, its reality. The eighty-one-year-old confused and incontinent woman whose delusion is that she is pregnant clings to what is to her a reality despite all objective findings to the contrary. For truth is objective and reality subjective. And as long as the latter is true, reality varies with the individual and is clear to anyone willing and able to interpret its meaning. What the old woman was saying was that she harbored within herself her own regressed self and was about to deliver it. If senility is the "second childhood," then she was pregnant with it and at the point of delivery. Viewed from this perspective her delusion makes sense, and her method of expressing it is poetry.

Fantasy building is a perfectly acceptable human activity, but its involvement in the construction of alleged historical sequences introduces an element of pure poetry or fiction that must be unacceptable to the scientist. At the same time scientists are often reluctant to reject such formulations altogether, if they are strung together in language compatible with scientific discourse. What I am doing is to defend speculative formulation, provided it does not pretend to any exclusive revelation, and remain attached to some documentary evidence.

Understanding the uniqueness of each person's reality, the young and the old, is the very essence of psychological skill—skill that must deal not only with the individual variance but also with the shifting and altering quality of this subjective state as the human being grows, develops, and ages. Each period in the life span of man forces on him a different reality, based on the altered physiology and the extent of the richness of the human experience. Old age can become an expression of the summation of human experience. It can be rich, varied, colorful, and in turn enriching; conversely it may be impoverished or empty and only serve to emphasize the futility of life and its meaning to many of the old. However, no matter what one's experiences may be, there is a need for an elaboration upon one's experiences, which tends to distort the objective truth but adds to the uniqueness of the reality that the individual wishes to convey. It is by far more real for it delineates more clearly to the observer the actual personality of the observed. It is more "real" of a personality structure of the communicating person than the actual facts warrant or state.

What emerges is a romanticized version of events; a dramatization of the facts; the good becomes magnificent, the sad—tragic. Again, a poetic interpretation of one's experiences in turn needs interpretation by the listener.

Furthermore, we who are engaged in the field of mental illness and health are quite aware of the permutations of time. We work with emotions that have their origins in the person's dim forgotten or repressed past but that make themselves ferociously felt in the present. No sooner does the patient express an emotion, a feeling, than it is immediately related to his past. Dreams know of no time dimension; past, present, and future permeate all three and operate as if the individual organism has no cognizance of that which we know as being temporal. What is needed most, therefore, in working with the emotionally ill elderly, is an understanding of their manifest behavior in the light of their lifelong experiences and affected as it may be by accrued deficits, both extrinsic and intrinsic.

Behavior is the aggregate of observable responses of the organism in its interrelationships. In its predictable form, it is the usual modality by which an individual handles life situations that may arise. It is usually automatic and reflexive, and more often than not it defines the character of the person. It is what one expects of one's contacts with another and upon which one projects a continuum of transactions. While minor deviations from the established patterns are allowed for, under certain circumstances, the usual set of expectations are those of stability, if not rigidity. Unfortunately, the predictability of behavior presumes a static quality of the source, the human being, who of course is in a constant state of change, development, and it is hoped, growth. Added to this dilemma is the subtlety of an ever-increasing spectrum of that which is called normal, due both to the greater tolerance by society of more and more deviant behavior and to the greater understanding that the helping professions bring to the study and alleviation of the human condition.

In view of the above, I have chosen to address myself to the psychodynamics of what I like to call agedness rather than aging. Aging is an ongoing process, therefore difficult of assessment. Agedness, however, is an assumed stance on the part of the organism that may or may not be due to organic dysfunction but may be behavioristically characteristic of a unified complex of roles, assigned, ascribed and much too often, acquired. It may be both character and pathology. It may be independent of any overt manifestations of organic disease and thus presents itself as a mode of coping or adaptive behavior most economical to the character structure of the individual. Behavioristically speaking, one may manifest agedness quite early in one's life, though usually it is characteristic of the later periods of the life cycle. Thus it is the manifest behavior of an individual that should interest us, and the latent meaning of its content that should intrigue us.

I assume that no one behavior is unique to a diagnostic category; therefore, individual symptoms are not reliable indices of a psychopathological grouping. Most studies on the psychopathological conditions of aging do not define etiological or pathogenic factors solely, and lacking such forces, such studies lead some of us to what may be described as empirical conclusions on behavioral patterns.

Perception-psychopathology relationships in old age is a case in point. "While some regard perception as an independent variable and direct our attention to the effect of disordered perception on personality development and consequent behavior, others view psychopathological conditions as independent variables and regard the perceptual behavior as outcomes or effects," writes Holzman. I, for one, am an adherent to the latter notion, having long since postulated the *exclusion of stimuli* in later life as an outcome or effect of a psychopathological if not psychodynamic condition.

"Perception, of course, refers to a perceptual act that transforms a physical stimulus into psychological information. Complex processes are involved in this transformation; reception of the stimulus, registration, the processing of the registered information, and the checking of the information against continued input. Eventually, the human organismal organization is meant to interpret all of the above in the light of its life experiences and effect action. Thus, sensory, cognitive, conceptual, affective and motor processes are all linked with each other in any given perceptual act." Most of us have long since recognized the crucial significance of perception, its central role in the development of those modulatory and controlling structures designated as the ego, or as I like to call it, the problem-solving self. For the perceptual act reflects the psychological point of contact between a person and the internal and external milieu. Its principal function is to convey information from the environment for integration with other psychological functioning such as memory, judgment, and anticipation. Obviously, too, it also receives and carries information about the nature and consequences of the perceiver's actions. Perception then is a central ingredient in effective adaptation, in the fitting-in process between the individual and the environment.

As the individual develops and moves toward active mastery, he/she can no longer depend on the instrumentality of others as in infancy, childhood, and adolescence but must amplify and coordinate the executive potential of his/her own body parts, which cease to be independent information and pleasure receptors and take up their collaborative, productive functions. In later life, owing to intrinsic and extrinsic vectors, recapitulation of early developmental sequences may take place, moving the individual from productivity to receptivity and in effect become dependent on the mastery or the instrumentality of others, an adaptive approach which in the belief of some is characterized by gross coercive dependence and/or by the disruption of proper ego functioning.

The threat of organ deficits or destruction within, the welling-up of heretofore unacceptable controlled impulses, and the all too frequent deterioration of the individual's socioeconomic status tax the adaptive capacities of the ego to the utmost. To master the threat of dissolution of its boundaries, to ward off any break with reality, the aging organism, having at its disposal a lowered psychic energy supply and being unable to deal with all stimuli, begins to exclude them from awareness. While of course the nature of the receiving organ obviously influences reception, many have carefully pointed out that perception is not a passive process. The physical stimulus is organized and transformed at the point of reception, and I like to believe that it never goes beyond the point of the sensory receptor.

The infant, too, is faced by the same problem of too many stimuli with little ego development to help it cope with them. However, the very young can and do take refuge in sleep or withdrawal to allow for a gradual exposure to the clamor, and the slow, measured, developmental integration of the stimuli and the evolvement of acceptable responses to them. Then, too, they have the help of supportive figures who are ever ready to supply ego judgment and strength to the struggling new organism. Both of these elements are not available, nor are they, only too often, acceptable to the aging individual, and hence the exclusion.

Though it may be argued by some that the mechanism of exclusion of stimuli is identical with the familiar mechanism of denial, it is my belief that this defense is rather different. Denial to me implies that a stimulus has been received, cathechted to, invested in, and then cathexis withdrawn. Not so with the exclusion of stimuli. It may be blocked at the point of entry, with a lowered threshold only for those stimuli relevant to one's narcissism, and, by the latter at this point, I mean survival value. The problem as one may see it is how to assess experimentally the rate and extent of the exclusion so as to utilize this mechanism as a psychobiological measure of aging.

As in all stages of the life cycle, cultural determinants substantially influence the variables of human behavior of the elderly. These patterns include not only moral standards and mores but also the more subtle patterns of motivation and interpersonal relationships. Variations in judgment and belief systems, such as religions and philosophies, are integrated with other cultural persuasions, such as child-rearing practices.

In the American culture, aged persons frequently are perceived as unattractive, unproductive, old-fashioned, useless, and querulous. These views are abundantly expressed and easily absorbed by youth. Thus, the values that a child accepts and incorporates with respect to elderly persons may emerge to the detriment in his/her self-perception in the late years of life. This built-in system of self-depreciation or denial may manifest itself in late life as inattention, withdrawal, irascible behavior, and so on.

One needs to examine the specifics of the value system of our culture to assess their influence on the elderly individual. According to Kluckhohn, there are five questions that each individual asks of himself throughout life, whether or not he is aware of it, and regardless of the level of his sophistication. Kluckhohn views this value orientation as: "A generalized and organized conception, influencing behavior of nature, of man's place in it, of man's relation to man, and the desirable and non-desirable as they relate to man's environment and interhuman relations." She states the questions as five problems that are crucial to all human groups: What is the character of innate human nature? What is the relationship of man to nature? What is the temporal focus of human life? What is the modality of human activity? What is the modality of a person's relationship to others?

The dilemma for the aged person may be illustrated by a brief examination of two of these: What is the human being's relationship to time? Which time dimension—past, present, or future—does a person value most? Clearly, in the American culture, healthy, active persons value the future. A substantial portion of the productive process is spent in planning for the future. Nothing is left to chance, not even a spontaneous good time. As the future becomes the present, it loses enjoyment; we are again planning for the future.

Yet old people, with little pleasant to foresee in the future, tend to be more concerned with the past. With a better tomorrow only a mirage at the twilight of life and a "future orientation" incorporated into their value system, the elderly are victimized by their own beliefs. Those who are younger have shunted them aside, if ever so subtly. Perceiving that they have relatively little time in the future, they tend to focus more attention on the past, but there is some pressure to do as much as possible in a limited time. Though old age is in a sense the twilight or Sabbath of life, some future time does remain.

Kluckhohn also acknowledges the need to identify the personality type most valued. Is it the "being"—the person most concerned with feelings, impulses, and desires of the moment? Is it the "being-in-becoming"—the one interested in the fullest realization of individual potential? Or is it the "doing"—the person directed toward action, achievement, and getting things done? The Mexican mother, oriented toward "being," may happily enjoy her child from day to day. The American mother, oriented toward "doing," will be fulfilled only as her child achieves. Achievement reflects her competence as a mother, an efficient manager, and a force in the community.

As long as an individual is "doing," he/she is integrated with the environment; as this process slows in later life, he/she is increasingly subject to extrusion. In old age, time for contemplation of life and its meanings is useful and healthy. But questions such as "What have I done? Have I reached the goals I set for myself?" must be approached with understanding that life is a series of compromises. Achievement is but one of the essential ingredients in the formula for successful living.

These are but a few of the elements that contribute insights, I believe, into the mechanisms involved in delineating the understanding of late life behavior. Insights into that which is injurious so as to help to alleviate pain.

Contributors

Fern J. Cramer Azima, Ph.D., Associate Professor, Department of Psychiatry, McGill University, and Co-Director, Therapy Day Center, Royal Victoria Hospital, Montreal, Canada.

Bertram S. Brown, M.D., Former Assistant Surgeon General, United States Public Health Service.

Mary Wanda Draper, Ph.D., Associate Professor, Department of Psychiatry and Behavioral Sciences, College of Medicine, University of Oklahoma Health Sciences Center.

Stanley J. J. Freeman, M.D., Psychiatrist-in-Charge, Social and Community Psychiatry Section, Clarke Institute of Psychiatry, and Professor, Department of Psychiatry, University of Toronto.

George F. Freemesser, M.D., F.A.P.A., C.S.B. Emmanual Convalescent Foundation, Aurora, Ontario.

James W. Fryer, B.S. Ind. Mgmt., Management Auditor, Community Services Division, Texas Department of Mental Health and Mental Retardation, Austin, Texas.

John Furedi, M.D., Ph.D., Director, Department of Psychiatry, State Central Hospital, Budapest, Hungary, and Mental Health Consultant to the Ministry of Health in Hungary.

Susan G. Himel, LL.B., Partner, Swadron, Brown, Cascone & Himel, Toronto.

Wayne H. Holtzman, Ph.D., President, Hogg Foundation for Mental Health, The University of Texas, Austin, Texas.

Robert E. Kogan, Executive Director, New Horizons, Clinton, Oklahoma.

Yvon D. Lapierre, M.D., Director of Research, Royal Ottawa Hospital, and Professor, Department of Psychiatry and Pharmacology, University of Ottawa, Ontario, Canada.

Heinz E. Lehmann, M.D., Professor of Psychiatry, Division of Psychopharmacology, McGill University, Montreal, Canada.

Ruth Ann Lyman, Ph.D., Director, Western Mental Health Center/Jefferson County Department of Health, Birmingham, Alabama.

N. Archer Moore, Ph.D., private practice, Macon, Georgia.

Domeena C. Renshaw, M.D., Professor, Department of Psychiatry and Director, Sexual Dysfunction Clinic, Loyola University of Chicago, Maywood, Illinois.

John T. Salvendy, M.D., Associate Professor, Department of Psychiatry, University of Toronto, and Director, Psychiatric Out-patient Services, St. Michael's Hospital.

William H. Simpson, Ph.D., Mobile County Community Mental Health Services, Inc.

Barry B. Swadron, Q.C., LL.B., LL.M., Partner, Swadron, Brown, Cascone & Himel, Toronto.

Jack Weinberg, M.D., deceased. Past Director, Illinois Mental Health Institutes, Professor of Psychiatry, Rush Medical College, Rush-Presbyterian-St. Lukes Medical Center, Professor of Psychiatry, Abraham Lincoln School of Medicine, University of Illinois at the Medical Center, and Distinguished Senior Scholar, Center for the Study of the Mental Health of the Aging, National Institute of Mental Health.